Improving the Mental Health Consultation

Improving the Mental Health Consultation

introducing a short circuit tool to aid patient understanding and dispel stigma

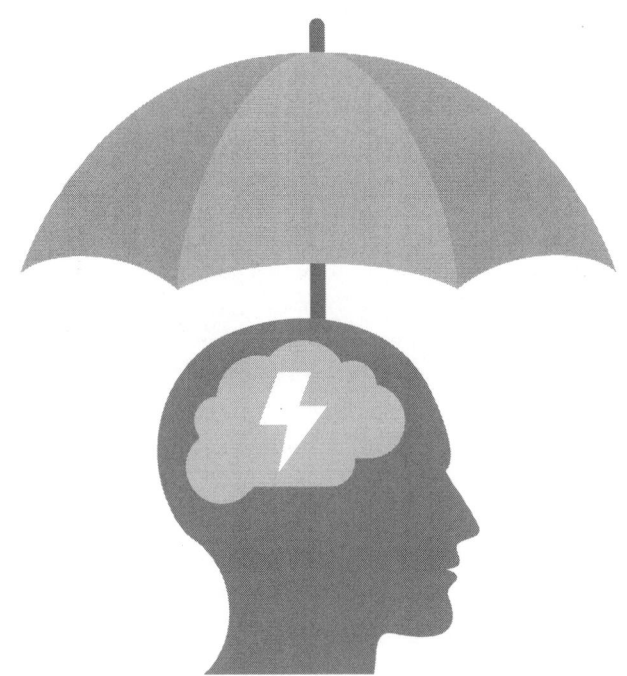

Shammy Noor

BSc (Hons) MBChB MRCGP PgCert Med Education
GP Partner, Darwin Medical Practice, Staffordshire

Scion

© Scion Publishing Limited, 2022

ISBN 9781911510970

A CIP catalogue record for this book is available from the British Library.

Scion Publishing Limited

The Old Hayloft, Vantage Business Park, Bloxham Road, Banbury OX16 9UX, UK

www.scionpublishing.com

Important Note from the Publisher

The information contained within this book was obtained by Scion Publishing Ltd from sources believed by us to be reliable. However, while every effort has been made to ensure its accuracy, no responsibility for loss or injury whatsoever occasioned to any person acting or refraining from action as a result of information contained herein can be accepted by the authors or publishers.

Readers are reminded that medicine is a constantly evolving science and while the authors and publishers have ensured that all dosages, applications and practices are based on current indications, there may be specific practices which differ between communities. You should always follow the guidelines laid down by the manufacturers of specific products and the relevant authorities in the country in which you are practising.

Although every effort has been made to ensure that all owners of copyright material have been acknowledged in this publication, we would be pleased to acknowledge in subsequent reprints or editions any omissions brought to our attention.

Registered names, trademarks, etc. used in this book, even when not marked as such, are not to be considered unprotected by law.

Typeset by Evolution Design & Digital Ltd, Kent, UK
Printed in the UK

Last digit is the print number: 10 9 8 7 6 5 4 3 2 1

Contents

Preface   vii
Acknowledgements   ix

CHAPTER 1 INTRODUCTION   **1**
    1.1 Mental health - the issue and a solution   1
    1.2 The global Covid-19 pandemic   7

CHAPTER 2 THE SHORT CIRCUIT THEORY   **11**
    2.1 'The short circuit' as a description of mental
         health disorders   11
    2.2 The symptoms of the short circuit   24
    2.3 The problem of insight   30
    2.4 The three Ps: personality, pressure and pathology 34
    2.5 The three Ps: patient assumptions vs. actual causes 39

**CHAPTER 3 THE SHORT CIRCUIT AS A TOOL: A PRACTICAL
APPROACH**   **53**
    3.1 Mental health presentations   53
    3.2 When to use the short circuit tool   56
    3.3 Using the short circuit tool in a
         consultation   67
    3.4 Summary   81
    3.5 Worked examples   82

CHAPTER 4 MENTAL ILLNESSES IN DETAIL   **85**
    4.1 Focus on anxiety   85
    4.2 Focus on depression   108
    4.3 Focus on OCD   141

CHAPTER 5 PHYSICAL ILLNESS WITH MENTAL HEALTH CONNECTIONS   **151**
    5.1   Focus on physical symptoms   151
    5.2   Fibromyalgia   160
    5.3   Irritable bowel syndrome   167
    5.4   Chronic pain syndrome   175
    5.5   Chronic fatigue syndrome   181

CHAPTER 6 TREATING THE PATIENT   **189**
    6.1   Management approaches   189
    6.2   Treatment modalities   196
    6.3   Dealing with pressure   202
    6.4   Cognitive behavioural therapy   208
    6.5   Pharmacological treatments   217

CHAPTER 7 SUMMARY   **257**
    7.1   Visualising mental illness   258
    7.2   Practical advice   259
    7.3   Mental health in detail   260
    7.4   Mental health with physical health   261
    7.5   Treatments   261
    7.6   Wrapping up   262

Preface

This book has been pitched to be both accessible and useful to a range of different clinicians who may be at different points in their career.

As doctors and nurses progress in their profession, they experiment with and learn different ways to explain and communicate complex ideas and concepts to their patients. There are as many different ways to do this as there are clinicians. The style used by any individual will develop with time and end up being a stamp of their own personality, both as an individual and as a clinician. Many times, patients may even choose their doctor on the basis of this style. We often call this our 'patter'.

The short circuit tool started with my patter. I used this patter often and found more and more success with it before deciding to develop it more formally so I could consistently use it with many different patients. You will have your own patter. For more junior colleagues, you may not yet have fully developed your patter. Maybe this book can help you do so.

The short circuit tool is fundamentally a way of describing mental illness to patients in a way that benefits both them and you. The book is divided into a number of parts:

The short circuit tool theory: you will first learn the theory of the short circuit tool and get a good idea of its concept.

The short circuit tool practical: you will then be shown how you can apply this in a consultation. Consideration will be given to when it could be appropriate to use the tool and how you would practically deliver the message to the patient.

Mental and physical health in detail: these chapters look in detail at the diagnosis and management of common mental health conditions. These chapters will be more like a traditional medical textbook. Each chapter refers back to the short circuit tool with an explanation of how this fits with and enhances the education of these topics.

Treating the patient: then there is a deep dive into the treatment of mental health conditions. The short circuit tool does not advocate one treatment method over another and is certainly not a method of treatment in its own right. It does, however, show the patient what is being treated and hopefully helps make whatever therapy option the patient takes more acceptable and understandable. A range of different options are explored and I would advocate that any clinician treating patients with mental health illness not only becomes familiar with, but masters these common treatment options.

Acknowledgements

This book would not have been completed without the support of many individuals in my personal and professional life.

I have been blessed to be working with the very best partners, staff and patients at my GP practice in Staffordshire, the Darwin Medical Practice. They have provided the ongoing intellectual stimulation and challenge which has inspired me to write my books. As a training practice in the West Midlands deanery we regularly get the brightest new GP trainees who keep us on our toes and they have been extremely helpful in tailoring this book toward the needs of the next generation of primary care clinicians.

The book was written entirely against the backdrop of the Covid-19 global pandemic, a period which has stretched every member of the NHS family. In the UK, primary care has been involved in not only the treatment of sick patients throughout the height of the various waves of the pandemic but also in the Herculean effort to restore normality through the vaccination programme. It does not surprise me one bit that our primary care institutions have coped admirably with this challenge and delivered the most successful vaccine campaign in medical history.

Despite this, many doctors, nurses and allied health professionals have taken an interest in my book and given helpful review material, and I would like to thank them for their time during this busy period.

Finally, the greatest thanks must go to my family – particularly my wife and two children. My kids have been without a daddy for too many weekends whilst I came home late from work and was locked away writing this book. I owe them a huge debt of gratitude and look forward to lots more weekends making up for lost time.

Chapter 1

Introduction

1.1 Mental health - the issue and a solution

1.1.1 The mental health consultation

I've been a GP for just over ten years now. During that time, as with so many other GPs, I have completed tens of thousands of consultations. Many of these have been linked to mental health – if the published statistics are to be believed, about a third of all of those thousands of consultations would be related. What I have learned over those years is that mental health consultations have a fundamentally different set of challenges associated with them. They have different patient expectations and perceptions. They are influenced hugely by the most nuanced and delicate use of language. They take so much longer and have so many factors that affect the outcome.

Of course, as medical professionals, we have a good understanding of the complex nature of illness and disease. We are not, after all, dealing with cars, which have a specific set of functions which either do or do not work correctly. Cars don't have predetermined beliefs about their own health, nor do they have individual needs and priorities. Nor do they have strong views on which tools they would or would not be prepared to have used on them. The straightforward questions are – does the car need fixing and can the car be fixed? Once the answers to these questions are established, the car doctor simply proceeds in the most appropriate way without much impedance.

No medical illness could ever be that simple. There is no blueprint for people, no manual or even a recommended set of criteria for what normal is. A human consultation will always have within it layers of complexity that would seem unimaginable to a mechanic. A rational plan of action, produced between doctor and patient, must encompass not only empirical science but also a complex mesh of biopsychosocial factors and emotional needs. This is true of the treatment of virtually any illness. However, illness of the mind sits significantly apart from others in this respect. It has some unique issues associated with it; issues which seem absurd in the context of other 'physical' illnesses.

These peculiarities seem to be mainly centred around stigma, belief systems and preconceptions. Take, for example, the very commonly heard phrase 'I'm not the sort of person who gets depression'. This does not seem to translate to any other form of illness – 'I'm not the sort of person who gets cancer'. This is not a phrase many doctors hear. 'My family won't believe me if I say it's anxiety' is commonly heard, whereas 'My family won't believe me if I say it's diabetes' is not.

The consultation for the patient with depression or anxiety, particularly in the diagnostic stages, can therefore be very complex and difficult – for both the patient and the doctor. These sorts of consultations often take much longer, require more emotional energy and can often feel less like there has been a tangible solution. This can be the case, for example, where the doctor believes there to be a diagnosis such as anxiety, but the patient does not. Patients in these circumstances feel that the doctor is not listening, whereas the doctor may feel that they cannot do anything for the patient, leading to frustration on both sides. Equally, where the patient and doctor come to different conclusions about the source of their mental health difficulties, the same frustrations arise. The doctor can often feel that they have nothing more to offer, whilst the patient is left feeling abandoned. No doctor wishes their patients to feel like this, so the consultation lasts much longer as both parties try to reconcile the situation by coming to a compromise solution – sometimes over many visits.

I, like others, have had many of these consultations. Like others, I had some successes and some failures in these circumstances. Sometimes the extra time and emotional energy resulted in a genuine improvement in a patient's health, and these encounters became a source of pride. Other efforts were failures – and these patients became the 'heart-sinks'. The term 'heart-sink' still very much resonates with me as a perceived failure. I would hope that there is something completely outside my control that has led to the heart-sink situation, but the niggling doubt would always be there that I had failed in my stewardship of the consultation to lead to this outcome. In reality it was probably a combination of many factors, some within my control, others not.

1.1.2 A change of style

What I did start to do, however, was experiment with different techniques, styles and methods. In particular, I tried to break the mental health mould by trying different ways to explain the illness.

> Phrases like 'admitting to...,' in association with mental illness, perpetuate its stigma as something to be hidden and ashamed of.

Some attempts were more successful than others. In particular I was interested in breaking down the stigma associated with those patients who I genuinely felt were suffering with depression, anxiety, OCD or some other form of treatable illness, but who held such strong beliefs about mental health that they wouldn't even entertain the idea of a diagnosis, let alone treatment.

Whilst on the subject of the differences between the medical consultation in mental health and other forms of illness, it is worth acknowledging the different language used by society, including medics, around the subject. The one term that often strikes me is 'admitting to' when describing mental illness. 'He needs to admit to the fact that he has anxiety'. Admitting to something has a connotation of wrongdoing – my son 'admits to' pinching the chocolate biscuits without asking, or a criminal might 'admit to' a burglary. One does not 'admit to' having asthma, or hypertension. Words like this, in association with mental illness, further perpetuate its stigma as something to be hidden and ashamed of. Patients often leave the consultation remembering specific words and phrases. These subtleties of language can, therefore, play a huge role in the ongoing belief held by the patient.

It is patently obvious to me as a physician that depression and anxiety are real and potentially serious conditions – indeed conditions with a very high rate of mortality in young adults. It occurred to me that to convince those patients, of whom there are very many who 'don't believe' in these things, a number of misconceptions would have to be challenged.

First among these was the fact that mental illness was not a feature of the patient's personal self or identity. 'How can I be depressed? I have always been the strong person in the family,' many patients say – which, on the face of it, seems logical, given a preconceived notion that mental illness is a function of inner strength. This appeared to me to be the foremost obstacle to the discussion about mental health. Some people with this belief would feel genuinely, and understandably, offended if their doctor suggested that depression or anxiety could be the cause of their problems. The consultation at this stage would become very tricky and take a long time, and the outcome would be variable! 'How can I have appendicitis? I have always been the strong one,' is a phrase heard significantly less often.

The other common misconception of mental illness is the association with life stressors. Clinicians will very often hear the phrase 'but I have nothing to be depressed about'. We know, of course, that life stressors will exacerbate and influence the relapse of mental illness, but they are not the only cause. Often patients can struggle with the notion that they should not be suffering because their set of life circumstances don't reach the perceived threshold of triggering mental illness. This can be torturous for some people. 'There are so many people worse off than me – I shouldn't be feeling like this,' they may say. This then adds guilt to their illness and worsens the course of their mental state. If they could see that stress and illness are related, but not the same thing, it would hugely help in the understanding of how they were feeling.

I tried a number of unsuccessful strategies to break the stigma. The most notable failure was the 'chemical imbalance' explanation.

The patient would fairly typically have held the notion that mental illness couldn't possibly be real, nor that they, of all people, could be suffering from such a thing. Telling such a person that this is, in fact, a real illness, featured by a certain 'chemical' present in the brain being out of balance, would often have no appreciable impact on them. Setting aside, momentarily, the current incompleteness of the neurotransmitter theories of depression, the 'chemical imbalance' perception for a patient is, in my opinion, inadequate. It raises many unanswerable questions. Hypothyroidism is an illness defined by an 'imbalance' of a hormone. This hormone can be tested. Its relative scarcity or abundance can be empirically and objectively determined. Once known, it can be corrected by either replacement of the deficient hormone or pharmacological blocking of excess hormone. The patient's symptoms improve, and a new test shows the balance is restored.

This treatment of an 'imbalance' bears no resemblance whatsoever to the diagnosis, treatment or follow-up of the depressed or anxious patient. This disparity does nothing to convince them that an imbalance is a good description of their illness. A patient would rightly ask, or at least think, that after treatment, their chemical status should be tested or monitored and would only feel reassured by the presence of the chemical within the 'normal range'. Since none of this happens, or indeed could happen,

> It occurred to me that to convince those patients, of whom there are very many who 'don't believe' in these things, a number of misconceptions would have to be challenged.

I think the patients would not feel any more enlightened by the description. Their preconceptions and health beliefs would likely remain firmly intact and any negative stigmas may even be reinforced by the lack of clarity. Furthermore, the term 'imbalance' feels somewhat loaded and potentially derogatory. 'The doctor said I was imbalanced,' a patient might take away. Clearly not the message that was given but very easy to inadvertently receive.

1.1.3 Developing the 'short circuit tool'

So, a new explanation of depression, anxiety or any other common mental health condition to the patient had to do a number of things. First, it had to satisfy them that this was a real illness, and not simply a function of being weak as a person. Secondly, it had to give them some concept of what this supposed illness actually is – what it does, and how it is different from simply having a certain emotion such as sadness or worry. And thirdly, it had to be able to show how this can cause symptoms, with or without stressful situations in life.

This where I found the 'short circuit' explanation came into its own. I started using this as a simple analogy of how thoughts in the brain might flow. It is not a theory, nor a literal explanation of what might be happening in the human mind. It isn't even a system or mantra. It is very simply a descriptive method to show how depression or anxiety might be affecting the mind. The power of this explanation is that it gives the patient a crystal-clear picture of why they are having the difficulties they are with their mental health. It also completely separates the illness process from their own personality, leaving them comfortable with the notion that they can still be 'strong' whilst suffering depression. It gives them a clear distinction between illness and life stress, whilst acknowledging the inevitable entangling of the two. And finally, it gives them clear hope that their illness can be treated, even if their life situation and stressors do not change. Clearly there is a strong belief amongst many depressed or anxious patients that the illness will never lift without the return of a lost loved family member, or the eradication of debt, or an improvement in their work situation. This belief can be stifling to the patient because in many circumstances, those life stressors may not have simple answers. Sometimes the doctor is the person least able to offer any real help to patients' life circumstances. This, again, can cause frustration to both doctor and patient as they begin to grapple with an unresolvable problem.

Over a period of time, I honed the 'short circuit' as an explanation and made it into a consistent tool that I could apply over and over again to many different patients who presented with a potential mental health condition but who could not entertain the idea of it affecting them – usually as a result of misconception and stigma. I found that by using the tool, patients were much more engaged with their treatments. Many exclaimed that this was the best way to describe what was going on in their heads. Many told their loved ones about it – and it often helped friends and family to see how mental illness is real. I am glad to say that many people are now successfully treated for their mental health condition. I think that without the short circuit tool they would potentially have remained ill for many years longer.

Following on from this wonderful feedback, I wrote my patient-facing book, *The Short Circuit*, published in 2016. I keep copies at the practice and a huge number of patients have read it, lent it to their loved ones and recommended it to others.

> The short circuit tool completely separates the illness process from patients' own personality, leaving them comfortable with the notion that they can still be 'strong' whilst suffering depression.

I use the 'short circuit' tool in my consultations many times per week. I use it often when first diagnosing someone with a mental health condition and when I review a new patient with a pre-existing condition that I have not met before. Patients would usually say that this was the first time they had seen mental illness described in this way. But often they would also say that they wished it had been shown to them before by other clinicians that they had consulted with. In 2020, I started to write this book to introduce the methods to any healthcare practitioner who has regular contact with patients with mental illness, and I have every confidence that at least some small part of this could find its way into the consulting methods of many clinicians.

1.2 The global Covid-19 pandemic

This book was written entirely during the global Covid-19 pandemic. At the moment of writing this, the vaccine has been rolled out to nearly four billion people across the world and in many countries a booster programme has started. Whilst infection rates are currently rising, certainly in the UK, the morbidity and mortality associated with Covid-19 is a fraction of what it was before the vaccination campaign. We sit in hope that this is the beginning of the end for the virus's grip on humanity.

The pandemic has affected virtually every person in virtually every country on the planet and in ways which we would have found unimaginable only a few months prior to the arrival of the novel coronavirus. Despite the advancement in healthcare and technology, one of the single key weapons in our armoury against infectious disease is the same thing that humans have endured in these circumstances for millennia – social distancing.

The pandemic has had a profound effect on mental health and wellbeing. This ranges from the mildest to the most severe end of the illness spectrum. In primary care, the proportion of consultations relating to mental ill health is about one-third. After about a year from the start of the pandemic, some estimates suggested that up to 60% of consultations were related to a mental health problem[1]. Even now, the mental health consultation rate is higher than prior to the pandemic. It is likely that this heightened prevalence of mental health problems in the population will continue for some time.

Covid-19 has had a number of direct and indirect effects:

- Coping with the direct effects of the disease – grief of mortality and of morbidity
- Fear of contracting illness in self or others
- Fears around accessing healthcare due to infection transmission
- Fear of long-term personal and social effects
- Isolation from work colleagues, friends and family.

Currently, the Mental Health Foundation is leading an ongoing, UK-wide, long-term study of how the pandemic is affecting people's mental health, working with the University of Cambridge, Swansea University, the University of Strathclyde and Queen's University Belfast.

---

[1] Bauer-Staeb, C., Davis, A., Smith, T. *et al.* (2021) The early impact of Covid-19 on primary care psychological therapy services: a descriptive time series of electronic healthcare records. *EClinicalMedicine*, **37:** 100939.

Near the start of the pandemic, a paper in the BMJ [2] concluded that "Increased psychological morbidity was evident in this UK sample and found to be more common in younger people, women and in individuals who identified as being in recognised Covid-19 risk groups", suggesting those with premorbidity were most affected. These findings have been confirmed in the long-term Mental Health Foundation study.

Similar to the BMJ study, the Mental Health Foundation [3] found that younger people (aged 18–24) report consistently lower coping levels than the general population, whereas older people (aged 55+) record slightly higher coping levels. It found that those with pre-existing health conditions remain the most at risk of heightened anxiety, followed by those with pre-existing long-term medical conditions. The rest of the UK population as a whole is also significantly affected, but less so.

Many people have adopted healthy coping strategies such as going for a walk and connecting with family and friends digitally. Some people cited limiting exposure to Covid-19 news and maintaining a healthy lifestyle as popular coping methods to deal with the stress.

However, unhealthy mechanisms were also being used by people to cope with the stress of the pandemic. In early April 2020, just after the first lockdown began, up to 20% of the UK adult population said they were drinking more alcohol as a way of coping with the stress of the pandemic; this rose during the pandemic to nearly 25% at its height but has since fallen back to 19%. Equally, many people (30%) stated that they were eating more than usual to cope with the stress of the pandemic. As with the figures for alcohol consumption, this rose (to a high of 40%) before settling back to about 30% at the time of writing.

---

[2] Jia, R., Ayling, K., Chalder, T. *et al.* (2020) Mental health in the UK during the Covid-19 pandemic: cross-sectional analyses from a community cohort study. *BMJ Open*, **10(9):** e040620.

[3] www.mentalhealth.org.uk/our-work/research/coronavirus-mental-health-pandemic

These changes to lifestyles may have a longer-term impact on the physical and mental health of the population for some time to come.

At the start of the pandemic, almost all of the focus was on the acute medical side of illness, such as assisted ventilation units and intensive care beds. Soon afterwards the mental health effects were being detected and discussed. Whilst the pandemic may have increased the overall level of the pathology of mental illness, it also had the dramatic effect of unifying the negative thoughts and concerns of patients. Patients with depression, anxiety or OCD, amongst other illnesses, were uniformly preoccupied with the same set of fears relating to the coronavirus.

Reassuringly, however, the Mental Health Foundation has found that the number of people 'feeling anxious or worried as a result of Covid' has significantly dropped in the latest round of surveys[3] (published February 2021). At the time of writing, levels of mental illness are still raised, both in prevalence and acuity, and it remains to be seen when, and if, these will return to normal.

The pandemic has also shown a side of humanity that is uplifting and enriching. There have been some positive side-effects of the change in human behaviour – such as a dramatic drop in pollution, traffic, infectious diseases and crime. There has also been a heightened awareness of neighbours, of the importance of healthcare and of the impact of mental health and wellbeing. We hope that these side-effects persist long after the pandemic has retreated.

Chapter 2

The short circuit theory

2.1 'The short circuit' as a description of mental health disorders

> **What you'll learn in this section**
> A basic concept of how the short circuit describes many mental health disorders, such as anxiety and depression.
>
> **How this helps**
> You will be able to appreciate these mental health disorders in a novel and simple way using an elegant visual 'short circuit'.

2.1.1 Introduction

Depression, anxiety, OCD and other mental health disorders commonly seen in primary care are defined primarily by the constellation of symptoms they produce. Depression, for example, is depression because it gives the patient a set of effects that can be described, qualitatively. Once a set threshold of markers is met, we call it depression. What this doesn't do is give the patient any clear idea of what the underlying pathology of depression actually is.

If we compared this to hypothyroidism, we see the difference starkly. Hypothyroidism gives the patient a set of symptoms – weight gain, tiredness, constipation and cold sensitivity, amongst others. But we do not define the condition based purely on the symptoms. We conduct blood tests and are able to pin down, precisely, a biochemical and pathological change which both explains the symptoms and defines the disease. Such a neat and well-defined pathological explanation, with an intuitively logical treatment set, does not exist for mental health disorders.

The 'short circuit' tool attempts to provide some form of intuitive description of the action of mental health disorders on the mind and more generally on thinking. In order to improve on the current situation of patient understanding, it needs to be simple and meaningful. If we can provide something to look at to 'see' the mental illness in the same way we can 'see' a thyroid function test result, this will dramatically improve the patient's view of their own illness and, by extension, reduce the stigma associated with it.

The 'short circuit' tool is an attempt to do just that.

The first thing to be clear about before going any further is that this is a tool for explanation. This is not scientifically established fact nor, obviously, any sort of literal representation of the flow of impulses through the brain. Its use in the patient consultation is not a diagnostic one, although there may well be occasions where you may feel this could provide evidence in forming a diagnosis. This section helps describe the short circuit and in further chapters I will discuss its use, as a consultation tool, in different scenarios.

Our brains are extraordinarily complex. In terms of interconnections, the human brain is the most complex entity in the known universe. Furthermore, neuroscientists are only just starting to grasp the basics of how this enormously complex mass of biological material can perform intelligent tasks almost instantaneously. It will be quite some time before anyone can claim to have completely understood the human brain and, despite the hype, true general artificial intelligence – the sort that makes the human mind so adaptable – is likely to be generations away.

Whilst the molecular biology and chemistry of brain tissue may provide some insight into the function of the mind, our knowledge is still very limited when it comes to higher level abstractions such as emotion and complex thought. The 'short circuit' describes the fundamental problem of depression and anxiety as a fault in this processing of complex thoughts. I have found this much more useful in helping a patient to understand than any attempt to describe chemical changes or dysfunctions of neurotransmitters.

In order to illustrate the short circuit, consider this patient.

> ### Case study - Lisa
>
> Lisa is a 45-year-old teaching assistant who is recently divorced from her husband and lives with her two sons. One is in his teens and has a diagnosis of obsessive–compulsive disorder, whilst the other is in his final year at primary school. The separation from her ex was bitter and traumatic but Lisa is proud of how she managed to cope and kept her sons well. She has been a keen table-tennis player for her local club but has in recent years found it difficult to find time for this. She recently lost her father, who after several years of battling dementia in a care home, died with pneumonia. Her workplace has been making some redundancies recently and she has concerns about her job security. Her older sister was diagnosed with breast cancer but is in full remission following successful treatment.

Let's consider how the tool describes what might be going on in this patient's mind.

2.1.2 'Normal thinking' - when there is no mental illness

First, you may have started to develop a picture of Lisa's life and personality. She has a variety of life stressors which will undoubtedly be giving her problems. We know that she has had a difficult marital split, she has the added pressure of mental illness in one of her children and she is naturally worried about her finances if she is made redundant. These life problems will surface in her mind, during the course of her day, as thoughts. These thoughts could be extremely varied; sometimes they will be about the past, sometimes the present or even about potential problems in the near or distant future. Lisa's thoughts could, at any one time, be about something small, something big and important or very trivial. Considering the almost infinite variety of human life and circumstance, these thoughts have an infinite variety. These thoughts are 'popping up' in all people all of the time. We all have these thoughts, some more than others and more at certain times in our lives than others.

Case study - Lisa

Lisa's thoughts might include:

- *'My house might be repossessed if I lose my job'*, or
- *'What have I done with my car keys? I won't get the kids to school on time'*, or
- *'I miss my father'*.

She may also have thoughts about more serious but less likely events such as:

- *'What if my child doesn't come home from school today?'*
- *'I'm so angry with my ex-husband I could do something I later regret'*
- *'What if I develop breast cancer and my children have to grow up without me?'*

The existence of all of these thoughts, no matter how serious or trivial, likely or unlikely, rational or otherwise, is entirely normal.

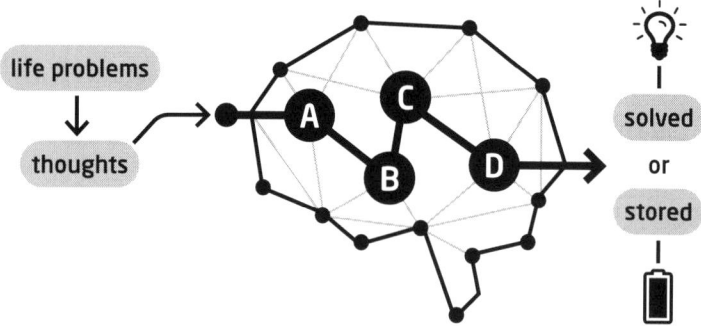

Look at the diagram above. This is a simplification but try to see this as how we would normally process a thought. It starts at point

A, moves to B then to C and D, etc. There is a logical workflow. The notion of moving from A through to D is, of course, purely metaphorical but provides a useful prop. When one of Lisa's thoughts that originate from a life problem pops up, it starts at the beginning of this journey. Think of A to D as a train of thought rather than four individual steps.

Under normal circumstances, the thought progresses along the logical workflow and reaches some form of end-point. This end-point might be that a resolution to the problem has been achieved – the problem is solved. Many issues will not have an immediate or obvious resolution, and in order for those thoughts to reach an end-point there needs to be a mechanism to store this to memory. These thoughts may surface again at some time in the future, but for now they have left the workflow from A through to D.

Case study - Lisa

Lisa, for example, may have the following train of thought:

- 'How will I get my work report complete when I have to take my son to his medical appointment?' ➜
- 'What if my work is thought of as substandard as a result?' ➜
- 'I will ask my deputy to cover some hours for me' ➜
- 'I will try to arrange my son's appointment at a time of day that minimises my time off work' ➜
- 'I will speak to my boss so she understands that my report may not be of its usual standard'

This thought has reached a conclusion and is therefore 'solved'.

However, some life problems are more difficult to solve, and thoughts associated with these may spend longer in the workflow. Often, when the thought comes to its conclusion, if it is not solved, it may be put in 'storage'. The thought will come back into the pathway when it next needs to be considered. This could be the following day, later that week or in the next year – depending, of course, on the nature of the problem at hand.

> ### Case study - Lisa
>
> Lisa may think:
>
> - *'My ex-husband was very wrong in the way he treated me and our sons'* ➜
> - *'Why did I let him get away with his behaviour for so long?'* ➜
> - *'Although we are now separated, it still hurts and makes me angry'* ➜
> - *'I have other things to do and think about today'*
>
> This thought has reached an end-point. The underlying issue is not 'solved' – the hurt of the past still exists – but the thought is 'stored' so that other thoughts can occupy Lisa's mind.

Different people may 'handle' these life problems in different ways. Different people have different levels of resources available to them in their lives which may make things easier – such as money or family. We have all experienced difficulties in life and we know that some people manage the life problem and the thoughts associated with these better than others. We all have different personalities and we all have individual outcomes to our thought processes. No two people will have exactly the same workflow to process thoughts; indeed, even in the same individual, the workflow might take a different path at different times in their life. This is all normal.

The thoughts themselves do not represent mental illness. There may be many more life problems and more thoughts at certain points in our lives, but no matter how many there are or what the nature of these thoughts is, it is not helpful to think of the thoughts themselves as part of the pathology.

2.1.3 Thinking with a mental illness

Now let's consider this altered diagram. This time the thought starts at point A and progresses to B and then C. However, now there has been a change in the workflow. From C, the thought gets 'short circuited' back to B. It then passes back to C, followed by B, then C, B, C, B. It can't get to its end-point. It's now stuck and the thought simply recirculates, persistently being batted back and forth from B to C to B to C. The affected patient will often have minimal control over this cycle. It doesn't matter what the thought is – there is the potential for it to get trapped. Thus the thought never reaches point D, after which it would have left the conscious flow and been either solved or stored.

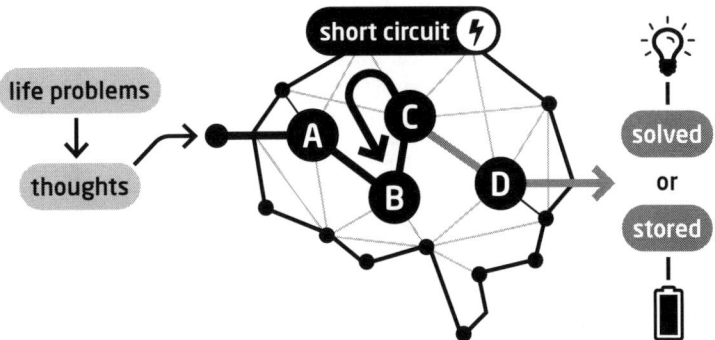

It is, of course, relatively normal to think about problems for a long time, regularly coming back to them. Different personalities will have different ways of doing this for their real-life problems. However, the key difference between a rational thinker who is voluntarily and deliberately considering a problem for a long time and someone with the short circuit present is that in the former, it is entirely under the control of the individual. They are able to switch it on or off at any time. With the short circuit, once the thought is bouncing between B and C, another part of the brain kicks in to try to stop the cycling. This 'back of the brain' is trying to tell the mind to 'stop it'. It is saying 'shut up', 'stop overthinking it', 'move on'. This dissonance between the short circuiting thoughts and the rational 'back of the brain' is key in the development of mental illness.

The existence of the short circuit itself indicates the presence of a mental illness. The patient is not actively looping the thoughts any more than an asthmatic patient is actively constricting their airways.

This short circuit description applies for depression, anxiety, OCD and a multitude of other mental illness. In the following sections I will break down how these differ. Suffering from one of these conditions, such as depression, therefore, is not the fact that life problems and the thoughts associated with them exist – we all have these, some more than others – but, in fact, it is simply the short circuit that causes the thought to be locked down into this cycle. Following this, an internal discord between the rational brain trying to break the cycle and the short circuit ensues. This simple, tiny fault is to blame for a vast array of outward symptoms.

The short circuit can be present in patients with many life problems, or in those with very few life problems. Equally the short circuit can be absent in those with many, or few life problems. The existence of the short circuit itself indicates the presence of a mental health problem. The patient is not actively looping the thoughts any more than an asthmatic patient is actively constricting their airways. It is outside their normal pathway of thinking.

This little loop could be described as the 'visualisation' of this form of mental illness – which as we shall see in further sections can include depression, anxiety or any number of related disorders.

Case study - Lisa

At various points in her life, Lisa has suffered with anxiety (and therefore the short circuit is present). At these times, Lisa's thought process may have looked like this:

- *'What if my son doesn't come home from school today?'*
- *'That's silly, he always comes home from school.'*
- *'But it's icy today, what if a car hits him and he doesn't come home from school?'*
- *'No, that's silly, but there have been kidnappings on the news.'*
- *'What if that happens to him, what if he doesn't come home?'*
- *'It is very icy; what if he is the unlucky one today and doesn't come home?'*

The thought is based on a life problem – and in its inception is a perfectly reasonable thought. Normally Lisa would process this A→D, reaching a logical conclusion. But now the short circuit is present, it bounces back and forth without progressing.

This little loop could be described as the 'visualisation' of depression, anxiety, or any number of related disorders.

In my experience of presentations of this looping effect, patients have immediately recognised and related to the explanation. 'Doctor, you have just nailed it, no one has ever explained it like that before'. I hear statements like this very often.

The short circuit can form the basis on which patients can start to separate the notion of mental illness from their life problems.

Once the short circuit is there, some thoughts can become stuck and cause symptoms. When the short circuit is not present, a patient with many life problems, in whom there has been a great deal of stress and pressure, will not suffer from mental health symptoms. It is, of course, perfectly possible for a patient to have a mental illness (short circuit present) at one point in their life and for them to suffer the effects of this, whilst at another time the short circuit is not present.

Many patients will be confused as to why at certain times of great life stress they did not have any mental illness, whilst at other times, where life problems were relatively small, they did. The short circuit helps explain this. When it is present, the mental illness exists, irrespective of the magnitude of life problems.

> ### Patient
>
> #### 'But I can't be suffering from depression, I have nothing to be depressed about'
>
> As you can see from the short circuit description, to suffer depression, the short circuit needs to be there. It can be there with or without 'life problems'. Hence the notion that depression can only exist with a 'reason' based on life stress, is not true. This does help break them into two separate entities, one with a causal effect on the other, but two entities, nevertheless. As the doctor, you can now point at a diagram and explain how these two things are different.

The thoughts that get stuck vary from person to person. These can range from incidents many years in the past, sometimes quite trivial, to major issues in the patient's life at the present time. When trying to treat a mental health disorder, it is extremely helpful not to get too side-tracked with the source of the problems themselves, because the treatment lies more in fixing the short circuit.

In the next section, I will describe how the nature of the thoughts that just stick in the short circuit determines the different type of mental illness the patient suffers – such as depression, anxiety, OCD and others.

> ## Patient
>
> ### *'So I can stop feeling this way – even though I can't change the past?'*
>
> Yes. This has now given the patient some hope. While it is common to believe that the only way a patient can be cured is for the problem itself to be solved, often the issue in their life may be completely unfixable or so far in the past that nothing can be done about it anyway. However, you can tell the patient that you can help to fix the short circuit. If you can get the workflow going again, no matter what the problem thought is, it will start to progress through to some logical end-point. That end-point may not be the complete solution to the problem but at least it won't be stuck and the looping will stop. Thinking will be more logical, more constructive and less all-consuming. This in itself can provide the patient with a huge degree of optimism and promise.

So now we are looking at mental illness in a new way. It no longer represents the magnitude of problems in a patient's life. Nor does it represent an individual's personality – anyone has the right to analyse thoughts in their own way. However, mental illness can be seen simply as the short circuit that exists in the thought-processing machinery. This is an illness, like any other illness. Just like asthma is a tightening of the airways, diabetes is a fault with the processing of glucose, or hypothyroidism is a depletion of hormone, so depression is a rational, demonstrable fault of an organ of the body – the mind. In the rest of this part of the book, I will outline how this simple, relatable description of the illness can explain a number of different symptoms and help the patient to recognise a range of issues.

I think patients' understanding is sometimes best advanced through analogy and I often use the radio analogy. Here it is in a nutshell:

> ## Consultation tip
>
> Try this explanation to your patient:
>
> *'Think of listening to a terrible news story on the radio. This can be a story that induces sadness, anger, fear or frustration. Now imagine the*

news story repeats itself over and over every 30 seconds. The radio itself is now stuck on repeat. The news story is now heard over and over. The emotion this induces is now magnified and can become overwhelming. It can be tempting to believe that the only way out is for the problem of the news story to be addressed in some way. This will of course help. But we must also fix the radio. If this is not done, then the next news story will become stuck and have the same effect over and over again. Fixing the radio does not, of course, change the news or the world. But it will allow the workflow to restart. The problem is still there but it does not cause the crippling symptoms it once did.'

The analogy takes minutes to explain but can leave the patient with a distinctly new view of the difference between life stressors and mental illness.

2.1.4 A note on the cause of mental illness

Key questions are: why is there pathology at all and what is the underlying nature of this pathology? Why does the short circuit exist in some people and not others? And in those that do have mental illness pathology, why is it there sometimes and not there at other times? These are searching and difficult questions, not least because there are no definitively established answers. I am personally asked this question often when doing mental health talks to groups of people from a wide range of clinical or non-clinical backgrounds. It is, perhaps surprisingly, only occasionally brought up by patients in the consulting room.

The search for a 'cause' for some people can be very emotionally consuming. It is a natural human trait to be curious to find reasons and the same applies to illness of the body and mind. The finding of a cause and the understanding of its nature can be empowering. Conversely those in search of these answers, who can't find them to a satisfactory level, can feel confused and powerless. The fact that medical science is unable to do this fully makes it ripe for many outlets, such as in social media, where many proclaim to have the answers to why mental illness exists and how to fix it. This can open vulnerable people up to financial exploitation and even abuse.

In some cases, patients can even turn away from treatments until they have found a convincing answer to the question of cause.

Patient

'I don't want any treatment unless I know why I am ill, and in any case if I have a medicine, it won't be treating the underlying cause.'

This is a particularly difficult place for the patient to be, given that current science can't answer the question with any degree of certainty and this answer is needed before any progress with treatment can be made. Patients can end up trapped in a cycle of mental illness without effective interventions. Furthermore, there are occasions where a particular stress-inducing person, place or situation becomes the sole target for 'blame' as the cause of a patient's mental illness. This, again, can lead to focus shifting away from effective treatment, whilst causing the patient's mental health to worsen as they grapple with an intractable stressful problem. The short circuit tool can be especially helpful here in separating pressure from pathology.

There are many common themes in mental health consulting – the issue of addiction to antidepressants, for example – but the fact that this very rarely comes up directly in a doctor–patient consultation is difficult to explain. I have used the short circuit tool many hundreds of times and found that once the patient has a good idea of what mental illness is doing to their thoughts, they are keen to move on to answer the question 'and what can I do about it?' Nevertheless, you should be able to give a concise and coherent answer if you are asked about the underlying cause of mental illness.

A fuller exploration of the current theories around the causes of mental illness such as depression and anxiety is given in *Chapter 4* under the relevant sections. This covers the biopsychosocial hypothesis which is currently the most complete model. A number of associated causes and contributory factors are also discussed.

Your patient may wish to go into more detail and you can refer to *Chapter 4* for more detailed explanations, but in a typical consultation where time can be limited, I feel you should try to cover the following in your answer:

Case study - Ameena

Ameena is a 43-year-old accounts clerk with three children who is going through a divorce and has had trouble with disruptive neighbours. She has recently started suffering the symptoms of anxiety. She asks 'I understand I am suffering from anxiety, but why is this? Why have I got it now? I want to get to the cause, not just treat something without knowing why it's there.'

The doctor's answer could include the following:

- 'There is, as yet, no definitive known cause for mental illness; however, we can try to identify triggers such as the stressful things going on at home.'
- 'There are certain things that might be considered "risk factors" such as the pressures in your life or your family history – but just as there are many people who have a certain risk factor, there are many that don't. No one factor is present in everyone and many people suffer anxiety even without any of the known risk factors.'
- 'Because medicines that affect the levels of certain brain chemicals can improve depression and anxiety, it is thought that these neurochemicals play a role.'
- 'Luck plays a big part in who gets ill and who does not – just like with cancer, anxiety can strike some people and not others.'
- 'Looking for a cause is natural but it is important not to spend too much energy doing this. It is highly unlikely that a single definitive "cause" can be identified in anyone.'
- 'Mental illness can be treated, and the treatments are often very successful, and sometimes life-changing. We should make sure we spend as much time looking for the right treatments as looking for a cause.'
- 'If you had asthma, even if we didn't know the underlying reason that you had the illness, you would still want the treatment so that you could be free of symptoms and live your life to the full – the same is true of anxiety.'

In the example above, it would most likely be very helpful to Ameena to be shown the short circuit tool to help her get an idea of how her anxiety is related to, but separate from, her life stressors.

2.2 The symptoms of the short circuit

> **What you'll learn in this section**
> An understanding of how, using the short circuit model, disorders like anxiety, depression, OCD and others are strongly related and are defined by the type of thought trapped.
>
> **How this helps**
> You will be able see how depression, anxiety and other related disorders are strongly interconnected and even share the same basic fundamentals.

I have often thought that maybe 'depression' needs to change its name. The word often conjures up so much prejudice and is associated with so much misinformation that it has become an almost useless term to use without thorough explanation. Not only that, but I'm not sure even once we get through the misinformation, that the word is a particularly good representation of what I have described in the previous section – perhaps 'thought process disorder' would be a better name.

But let's consider what the effects of this thought workflow error are. Consider a patient whose thoughts are locked down; thoughts about life problems never get past point C and are left bouncing from B to C to B to C. Many people who suffer with a range of common mental health problems can relate to this. Hours go by and the same thought may be swirling around and around. Then another thought may appear at point A. This too may never reach point D, forever trapped between B and C. People will sometimes realise this is happening. A 'back of the brain' inner voice will appear, saying 'stop it, stop going over this again and again'. This inner voice may succeed for a period of time but after a while the thoughts will reappear, start at point A and get trapped in the cycle again.

In the same way that you can point at a radiograph and say, 'this is a fracture,' you can now point at a diagram and say, 'this little short circuit is the cause of your mental health symptoms'.

Now the patient's brain is giving a disproportionately large amount of energy and time to this process. The thoughts become like bees, buzzing in the head, unremittingly, and so it becomes more difficult to concentrate. When trying to engage in conversation with other people, there is a constant distraction, and irritability and anger often develop. Things which would normally be enjoyable no longer are – how can you enjoy your favourite TV show, a round of golf or your time with grandchildren, with the unrelenting buzzing in the brain? Furthermore, sleep is disturbed and fitful and many people find themselves awake early in the morning when the buzzing begins again. These are all the effects of the short circuit on the brain's ability to do all its other jobs. And as a result, all of these other jobs suffer.

You can now start to see the link between the simple visualisation of the illness and the range of symptoms. In the same way that as a doctor you can 'point' at a set of abnormal blood results and say 'this is diabetes' or 'this is hypothyroidism,' or you can point at a radiograph and say, 'this is a fracture,' you can now point at a diagram and say, 'this little short circuit is the cause of your mental health symptoms'.

But this is not all. The nature of the trapped thought itself is important. You may have noticed that at points in this book I have used the term 'common mental illness' – using depression, anxiety and OCD, amongst others, interchangeably. In fact, these syndromes share the exact same cause when you look at the short circuit.

Many mental health disorders, such as depression, anxiety and OCD are defined by the syndromic set of symptoms they produce in the sufferer. The short circuit differentiates them in a useful but slightly different way which helps the patient understand how these seemingly different disorders have so much in common. This differentiation is related to the type of thought that gets trapped in the cycle.

In the same way that you can point at a radiograph and say, 'this is a fracture,' you can now point at a diagram and say, 'this little short circuit is the cause of your mental health symptoms'.

2.2.1 Nature of the trapped thought

All of these mental health disorders share the short circuit as the key feature but small differences in the type of problem thoughts that are locked in produce different outward syndromes, such as depression or anxiety. See the table below:

Type of life problem	Nature of thought stuck	Disorder
Past or present problems – things that have already happened	'how come?', 'why?'	depression
Future possibilities – things that might happen	'what if?'	anxiety
Incomplete task – things that need doing or achieving	'have I done…?'	OCD
Specific traumatic event – e.g. an assault in the past	flashbacks of event	PTSD
Body image – e.g. weight or looks	'my body looks wrong'	body dysmorphic disorder, eating disorders

When the looping thoughts are about things that have already happened – either in the past or in the present of the patient's life, they get symptoms characteristic of depression. In those suffering with anxiety, the problem thoughts are about bad things that may happen in the future. The underlying problem, the error of processing, is the exact same short circuit that prevents thoughts from progressing through the workflow in a productive and rational fashion. When the locked thought is about an unfinished task, the outward symptoms are those characterised by OCD.

You can now start to show the patient how depression, anxiety, OCD and other common mental health problems are strongly linked. Patients are often perplexed as to which diagnosis they have and why their symptoms often cross multiple diagnosis types. This lack of clarity in the patient's mind can be extremely difficult to live with.

However, once patients have been shown that the existence of the short circuit is the key pathology, it becomes much easier for them to see that they can easily have part depression, part anxiety, part

OCD or another short circuit-type syndrome. This is also helpful, as discussed in other sections, in explaining why the same medicines and therapies can be successfully used, almost interchangeably, with any of these conditions.

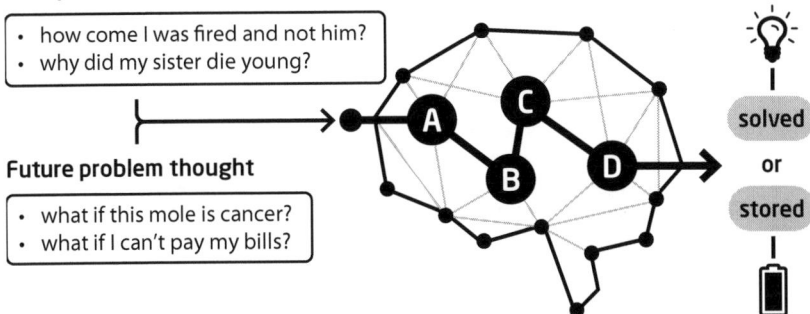

Past problem thought

- how come I was fired and not him?
- why did my sister die young?

Future problem thought

- what if this mole is cancer?
- what if I can't pay my bills?

Look at the diagram above – this might be an individual with a number of life 'stressors'. These are the things that appear in their workflow. Whilst there is no short circuit, all of the thoughts about these life problems occupy the person's brain for a finite, proportional amount of time and end with either some resolution of the problem or some mechanism for that thought to be stored so the mind can be used for its other necessary functions.

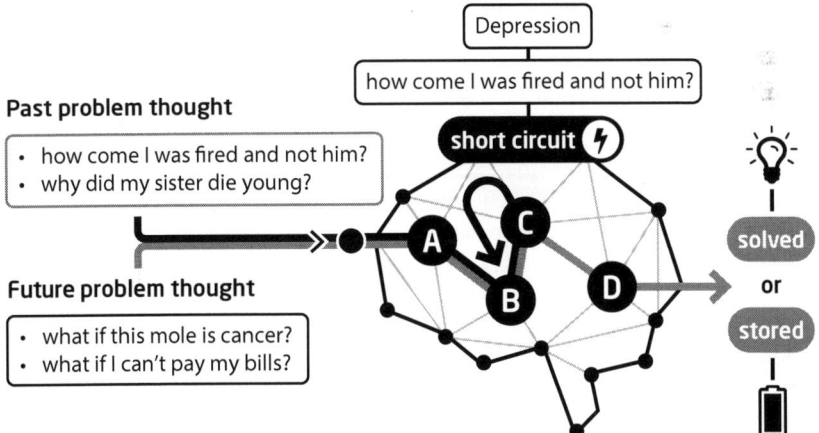

Past problem thought

- how come I was fired and not him?
- why did my sister die young?

Future problem thought

- what if this mole is cancer?
- what if I can't pay my bills?

However, take an individual, with the same life stressors, who now has the short circuit present. As you can see in the above diagram, some of this person's thoughts progress through from A to D, eventually leaving the brain solved or stored, whilst others are thrown off track by the short circuit and end up trapped. Here, past problem thoughts are getting trapped, whilst future problem thoughts are passing through. It may be work incidents haunting them from the past or even the most trivial issues in their lives now.

Section 4.2: Focus on depression will explore this form of short circuit disorder in more depth, but you can see, fairly logically, that this person who is thought looping about a bad event that has already happened will have a feeling of sadness. They may feel angry or personally hurt. The range of emotion associated with depression is vast and may include loneliness, insecurity, hopelessness, futility of future actions and damaged self-worth. When people experience depression and thoughts are bouncing about a problem that has no obvious solution, such as a bereavement, it can feel as if the situation has no resolution. How can they ever feel better unless their loved one comes back? How can they get out of this loop whilst they are still being bullied at work? Not only is this mentally exhausting, it is physically draining too. Depression is one of the biggest causes of persistent unexplainable fatigue and doctors will recognise it as a cause of TATT (tired all the time). Again, the short circuit helps the doctor explain to the patient why this connection is there and provide reassurance that by addressing the short circuit, their symptoms will improve without having to necessarily change the life stressors.

Once the short circuit is fixed, the life problems will still be there and the thoughts will still appear; however, they will flow and not get trapped. There will be relief.

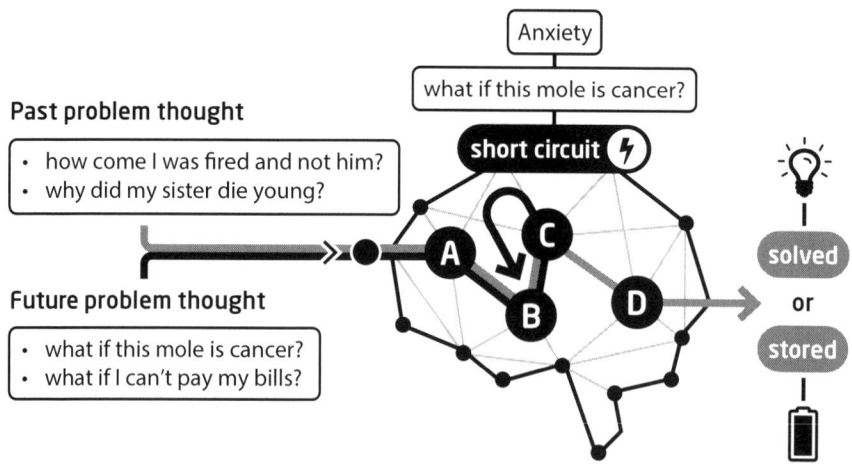

On the other hand, consider if the patient's looping thoughts are about something bad that may happen in the future. 'What if my son doesn't come home?', 'The plane might crash' or 'What if this mole is cancerous?' This person will be nervous. They will be afraid and panicked. They will be obsessive about trying to stop the bad events from playing out. They may be extra vigilant and wary. They may have some of the same features of the person suffering with depression – they may feel angry, insecure and out of control. But the overall physical manifestations of those suffering predominantly with depression compared to those with anxiety may be remarkably different. And this is probably the reason that the two illnesses are not often considered by patients together but, as has been explained, they share the very same underlying core issue as viewed through the lens of the short circuit.

However, with just a little change in the character of the problem thought that gets trapped, the effect further downstream can be huge. Like depression, anxiety can also be associated with a number of symptoms affecting various organs of the body. Since anxiety is much more likely to invoke an adrenaline-mediated *'flight or fight'* response, the outward physical symptoms are vastly different. The heart beats faster; palpitations are felt; breathlessness can be experienced. Many patients describe the sensation of pins and needles in their fingers and toes. On top of this, the physical symptoms themselves can start a new trapped thought – 'What if these palpitations are the sign of a heart attack?' This can further exacerbate the problem – this is known as secondary anxiety. It is clearly understandable that patients might assume these symptoms are cardiac in origin. I often describe this to patients as 'the mind races, then the heart races, then the mind races in a vicious circle'.

> With just a little change in the character of the problem thought, the effect further downstream can be huge.

Section 4.1: Focus on anxiety will consider in more detail the specific features of anxiety and the phenotypic differences between anxiety, depression, OCD and other common disorders which share the same underlying 'short circuit' explanation. We will consider how and why their physical manifestations can be so different despite sharing such a similar fundamental 'error' – the existence of the short circuit.

Once the short circuit is present, patients could describe symptoms of depression, anxiety, OCD, PTSD, eating disorder or others. In some it can be a roughly even split of two or more conditions, whilst in others it is predominantly one or another. Whilst the physical manifestations may be different, there really isn't much distinction to be made. They are really just different forms of the same thing. You can see, therefore, that with a simple explanation of the short circuit tool, patients can understand that depression is 'thought bouncing' for an event that has already happened and anxiety is 'thought bouncing' for a possible future event. This makes it much clearer to a patient how the two are linked.

This does a great deal to help patients who desperately struggle with the notion that they ought to have one diagnosis or another – but seem to have both. 'One doctor says I have depression, whilst another says it's anxiety'. It does a great deal to help patients understand why they have been given an 'antidepressant' – even though they have OCD symptoms and do not display the typical symptom set of depression. These patients all have the presence of the short circuit. They each have different types of thought that get stuck, some with multiple types. In later chapters we will discuss treatments which fundamentally help the short circuit, and therefore are effective in all of these forms of mental health disorder.

2.3 The problem of insight

What you'll learn in this section
An understanding of how insight is blunted in common mental health conditions.

How this helps
By recognising that both patient and society can have limited insight into mental health conditions, it can help you understand your patients' perspective.

There is another peculiarity about treating patients with mental illness compared to other forms of illness: the potential loss of insight. This illness can itself sometimes make the patient believe that they do not have it. Mental health problems can present in many different ways and this is discussed in *Section 3.1: Mental health presentations*. Many GPs will be familiar with the ICE consultation model which suggests the clinician explore the patient's ideas, concerns and expectations. Whilst some patients will have insight into the possibility of a mental health problem as the cause of their symptoms, others will not. For example, the ideas of a patient with palpitations in whom there is a lack of insight, will often not include, for example, anxiety as a possible diagnosis. Their concerns will more likely be skewed towards excluding a cardiac diagnosis and the expectation may be to be referred to a cardiac specialist.

There are many examples in the biology of viruses or bacteria that, once they infect another organism, go about making changes to the host that dampen its ability to detect the invader. In terms of evolutionary biology, this is great for the attacker.

I find the similarity of mental illness to the actions of microbes and other biological phenomena somewhat interesting. Consider HIV, a virus that owes its success, in part, to the fact that it attacks and destroys the very system in the body that would detect it and remove it. In essence, the body's own immune system eventually fails to recognise the virus, which does a very clever job of hiding itself. On a cellular level, the virus has dampened the insight of the body's defences, which no longer see it as foreign, abnormal or dangerous – they can't even tell whether it is there or not. This tactic of switching off the host's ability to recognise the virus as different is very effective, and there are many subtly different ways in which this can happen.

Larger organisms will do this too. Consider the mosquito. At best, it's an annoying biting flying midge; at worst, it is the vector for one of the biggest causes of death in human history – malaria. When it lands on the skin of its prey it injects saliva through its proboscis which contains immune material that can give the *Plasmodium falciparum* parasite a sort of invisibility to its host.

Depression, anxiety and other forms of illness of the mind can often reduce a person's insight. OK, they are not viruses, nor insects – but they do trick the victim's mind into invisibility. There aren't many illnesses like this. When you have pneumonia, you know you are ill. There's no mistaking the pain of a heart attack or meningitis or an epileptic seizure. But when the disease is of the mind, very strange things can happen. It becomes harder and harder to know the difference between a thought process that has been created or moulded by illness and another one that is normal and real. This can be very stark in the more vivid disorders like schizophrenia.

As a clinician, if you see a clear phenomenon such as 'delusion of reference' where the patient believes that a news story on television or in a newspaper is about them specifically, the loss of insight is very clear. In the medical profession we are often frustrated by the lazy portrayal of mental illness in the media and film. Schizophrenia is a typical example of one which is commonly misrepresented as some form of dual personality. A very good counterexample, however, was the superb film *A Beautiful Mind*. In the opening sequences, we see the protagonist, the Nobel laureate John Nash, involved in a tense stand-off between US Department of Defense special agents and Russian spies. It's gripping and the audience is wholly engrossed. It's only later in the film we realise that the entire set of events is delusional, but up until that point we would have no way of knowing that it was anything other than the absolute truth. Thus the film portrays a more accurate representation of schizophrenia. I will allow the fact that in the film, the hallucinations are incorrectly presented as visual rather than auditory, as artistic licence – an auditory hallucination would be difficult to portray on screen!

These are somewhat extreme examples. In the more common illnesses of depression or anxiety, the same invisibility can occur, even if it is not so dramatic. I think this is a particularly important concept to grasp in the mental health consultation. It fundamentally changes the dynamic of the process when the patient has no insight into the fact that a disabling illness of the mind could be responsible. It is very important too, to understand that this is not a feature of the intelligence, personality, education or demographic of the patient.

You could say that the patient's brain is lying to them or that they have failed to understand. I do not believe this is the correct way to think of this. The illness lies. And the illness protects itself by making itself invisible and making the brain believe that the abnormal thoughts are real. Where other people around them may see that their thoughts are changed or more irrational, they themselves may not see it. This is not because they are not intelligent enough nor because they haven't thought it through, but because the illness has in some way protected itself by reducing the person's insight. In depression, the feeling of hopelessness or worthlessness can be overwhelming. In fact it is a lie. The illness is talking and when the patient is better – only when the patient is better – will it become obvious that this was a lie all along.

> You could say that the patient's brain is lying to them or that they have failed to understand. I do not believe this is the correct way to think of this. The illness lies.

Unfortunately, it doesn't stop there. Whilst the patient's insight is blunted so, it seems, is the insight of society as a whole. It is an unfortunate combination that an illness almost invisible to the sufferer also blinds the community in which the sufferer lives. How can people believe in the invisible, untouchable, 'non-physical' disease any more than they can believe in fairies? A person with a leg amputated is clearly suffering from a disability – you would be hard pressed to find disagreement with that statement. But far too often and for far too long, those disabled with illness of the mind are not given the same support. What some people see is not an illness but a person who is simply angry, withdrawn, confused or hapless. The inclination is to blame the individual for having a weakness of their personality or mental constitution. The knee-jerk reaction is to want them to stop being lazy and 'pull themselves together'. Once again, the devil that is the disease escapes any form of scrutiny or challenge. And again, I would say that the solution to this involves the 'visibility' of the illness.

Mental illness seems to occupy this almost impossible position of blinding the sufferer and being ignored by society through the disbelief in its very existence.

As the patient's clinician, it is important to have a good grasp of this potential lack of insight. Insight can be a very tricky thing to bring up in a consultation. It can be very difficult to describe and by its very nature, would require the patient to take a leap of faith to believe that what their mind is telling them may not be the whole truth.

2.4 The three Ps: personality, pressure and pathology

What you'll learn in this section
A number of factors contribute to a personal emotional state and in this section, I introduce the concept of the three Ps.

How this helps
You can now understand how these three separate but connected entities can be broken down, metaphorically, to help understand the cause of a patient's emotional state.

2.4.1 Introduction

We have described depression, anxiety or any related mental health disorder as fundamentally a disturbance of thinking. This is in the same sense that diabetes is a disorder of the endocrine system and pneumonia is a disease of the respiratory system.

Before we can begin to treat patients with a disease of a bodily system, we usually try to understand the system itself – in the case of mental illness, the brain. Of course, there exist numerous disciplines, each concerning a different aspect of this overall understanding. Anatomists, for example, are interested in the physical form of the brain, whilst physiologists wish to understand the physical functions themselves.

But how will we go about defining and understanding 'thought'? This is a much more elusive and difficult task than, say, the study of the kidney. The anatomy of the organ of thought – the brain – is well described; however, we are probably still many generations away from having a comprehensive theory about how this anatomical form produces conscious thought.

A huge amount of time and effort has gone into trying to understand thought, and its physical and metaphysical origins, processes and effects. Academic disciplines as wide-ranging as psychology, neuroscience, philosophy, artificial intelligence, biology, sociology and cognitive science have been involved. Thought underlies many human actions and interactions. It allows humans to make sense of, interpret, represent or model the world they experience. It allows us to make predictions about that world and mould it. To humans, who have needs, objectives, desires and plans, thought is perhaps the single most important life-sustaining process.

There have been many advances in all of the fields described above, each edging us ever closer to the ultimate goal of a fully inclusive theory and understanding of the brain, consciousness and thinking. Of course, we only have the human brain as the fundamental tool of intelligence – it will remain to be seen whether it is indeed powerful enough to understand itself.

Since we will be unable to be very precise about what we mean by 'thinking', an element of abstraction and simplification is necessary – especially when it comes to a short interaction between clinician and patient. For our purposes, we do not need to fully grasp the complex shape of the brain nor the underlying mechanisms of how it works. We are interested in the end product – the thought, the feeling or the idea. Remember, this is about helping a patient suffering from a mental health condition, in your consultation. It needs to be quickly understandable, easily and quickly deliverable and immediately impactful. The exact physical nature of thought is unknown and in essence is likely to remain unknown for a long time. Nevertheless, it is still immensely useful to categorise and describe the behaviour of thoughts and thinking with a view to understanding the cognitive process, if not the biological or chemical.

From the short circuit tool, a beautiful realisation comes out. It visually and conceptually helps discern three elements that influence a patient's thoughts. This can be fundamentally helpful to both clinician and patient in determining the most helpful course of action to follow. I call these the three Ps:

- **Personality**
- **Pressure**
- **Pathology**.

2.4.2 Personality

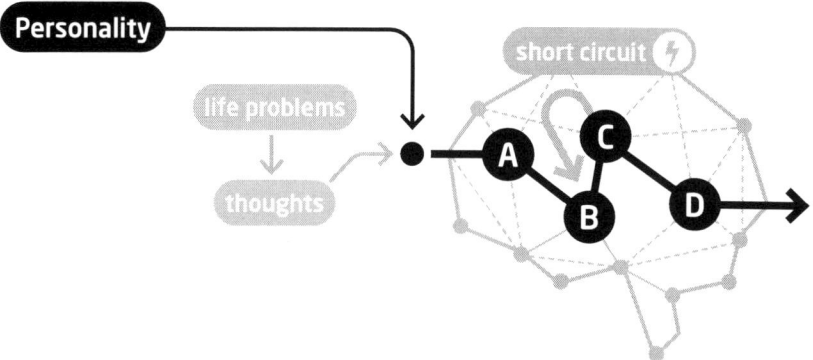

Relating to the short circuit diagram, personality can be seen as the way the thought flow processes A through to D are connected. This will be different in different people – in fact will be unique to the individual. In this description, personality is separate to illness and fundamentally separate to life problems. This metaphorical 'route' of thinking from A to D may be somewhat under the control of the individual and in many respects might even define their individuality and sense of self.

2.4.3 Pressure

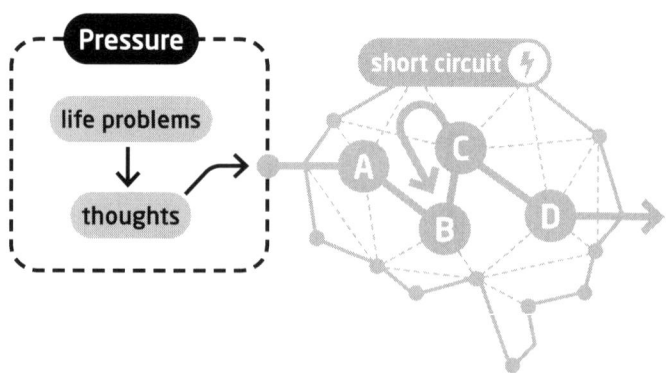

Pressure, in the diagram, is represented by the 'traffic' flowing into and through the pathway. Under heavy load, a person's thought flow will be filled with numerous thoughts, ideas and emotions. Imagine your patient had problems with work, money or a relationship. These life problems will present with thoughts which are more numerous and occupy a great deal of 'resource' for the brain. Again, this is a separate entity to the existence of illness and personality. Any combination of personality and life pressure can, and does, exist.

2.4.4 Pathology

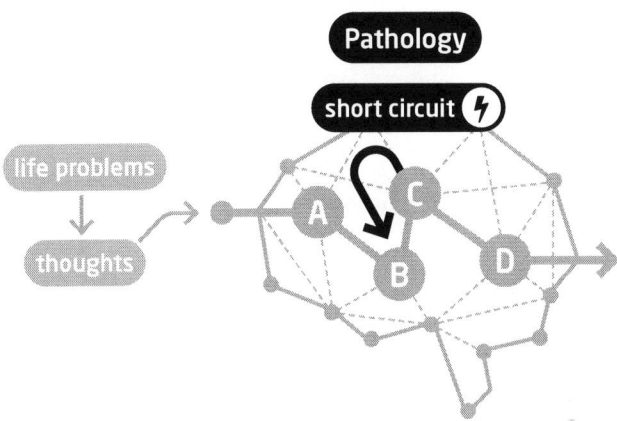

Pathology is a different thing. Pathology, as seen in the diagram, is the loop that appears between B and C. As I have stated previously, this is not a literal description of anatomy, physiology or histopathology. However, as a descriptor of anxiety or depression and as a 'visualisation' of an invisible illness, this is extremely powerful.

I have shown this very diagram to hundreds of patients. The reaction has been almost unanimous. Patients who have depression or anxiety have exclaimed that this is the best representation of what is going on in their head that they have ever seen. Many patients have said that the penny has finally dropped. It has in very many cases almost immediately transformed people's understanding of depression from a 'made-up' entity to a real-life condition that they can fully identify with.

With this simple description, it can clearly be seen that personality is fundamental to the individual and pressure is explicit, and there may or may not be much you can do for the patient as the clinician. But the third P, pathology, is illness and can be actively treated. The illness of depression or anxiety will start to have effects on emotion and thinking.

Many patients are unaware of the existence of the third P, and they might attribute their thinking to the other two Ps. Therefore they might attribute the problem to their personality and tell themselves, 'Pick yourself up and snap out of it!' Such patients may also look at the level of pressure they are under and conclude that they should not be thinking like this with that particular level of stress, telling themselves, 'Come on, there are people out there with much worse problems than you'.

Very quickly, it becomes much easier for the clinician to show that mental illness is a distinct entity, and the diagnosis and treatment of it is not a reflection of the individual's personality. This is immediately better for a patient to comprehend and handle. Often when the patient is consulting for the first time about a mental illness, they have spent years wondering what aspect of their own personality needs changing to stop the symptoms – often this exercise will have been in vain. Since we are now presenting pathology and personality as two separate and distinct entities, it can be seen that the short circuit can affect any personality type – shy, extrovert, strong, lazy, rational, analytical, etc.; just like cancer.

Apart from separating personality from pathology, the other very useful advantage of the short circuit tool is the separation of pressure and pathology. Some patients will be confused by the lack of direct correlation between life stressors and the symptoms of illness. Whilst it is well recognised that life events can trigger or significantly magnify mental health problems, there are many occasions when the two do not necessarily go hand in hand. Patients will say 'But I have nothing to be depressed/anxious about' or 'But I went through a horrible divorce a few years ago and didn't get any of these symptoms'.

> The short circuit can affect any personality type – shy, extrovert, strong, lazy, rational, analytical, etc.; just like cancer.

Other patients will say that the mental health condition is so intricately linked with the pressure that they are effectively the same thing. 'My anxiety will be entirely resolved once my housing situation is improved'. Of course, if anxiety is present as pathology, it is likely to have predated the housing pressure of this patient and may continue after the housing situation improves.

Many doctors will argue that they can't do any more for a patient unless the patient's life pressures change. This may or may not be true; in fact there are a number of interventions that a doctor can usefully make to impact on the patient's 'pressure'. These are discussed in *Section 6.3: Dealing with pressure.*

However, for most clinicians, given the skill sets and resources we have at our disposal, we must do everything we can to address the third P, pathology, through intervention. The interventions, which are discussed later, could be behaviour changing, talking therapy or medicinal.

By introducing the short circuit (described as a tool in *Chapter 3*) to the consultation, it becomes relatively clear to the patient that pressure and pathology, being separate things, can exist one without the other. When a patient has the short circuit present then any thought process can become stuck in the loop, without there being a huge and obvious stressor. Equally, patients can be going through a huge amount of personal stress but not necessarily getting symptoms of mental illness. The worst case scenario, of course, is to have both.

2.5 The three Ps: patient assumptions vs. actual causes

What you'll learn in this section
Patients' ideas and assumptions about the cause of their symptoms may differ from the actual cause, with the three Ps being confused with each other.

How this helps
You will be able to recognise nine different scenarios which match the patient's assumption with the actual cause of emotional symptoms.

2.5.1 Introduction

In the previous sections, I have described the differences between emotional symptoms arising from personality, pressure and pathology. With these three entities separated, it is useful to consider points in the consultation where patients may have a preconception (and possibly a misconception) of the cause of their mental health symptoms.

The personality represents the nature of the person. This could be naturally shy or extrovert, impulsive or reflective, worrisome or carefree, or in fact any one of an infinite range of possible combinations. The pressure represents the combination of stressors in a person's life. These will usually be listable and often tangible, but not always. The reaction to the pressure will depend on the personality and although it will often be rational, it may vary in different people and at different times.

Pathology is the existence of a mental health problem – in this description, the short circuit. This will, of course, present itself as mixed with the personality and the pressure, but is a distinct entity for the purposes of this illustration.

Patients will arrive with ideas about the underlying cause of their symptoms. A detailed discussion of the symptoms of the common primary care mental health presentations is given in *Chapter 4: Mental illnesses in detail*. In the case of mental illness, patients may attribute pathology to personality or pressure.

2.5.2 A patient example

Case study - Daniel

Daniel is a young chartered accountant, who, having recently completed his training and exams, is now working in a medium-sized firm. Whilst extremely pleased that he was successful in his accountancy exams, he is finding the work stressful and tiring and resents the way he has been treated by some colleagues. He has recently split up with his long-term girlfriend and has moved back in with his parents. He is looking for a new flat to live in as the commute from his parents' home to work is very long. He has found himself in numerous arguments, getting angry and upset and sometimes shouting. He later regrets his actions but is constantly worried he will do something that will lose him his job and cause future financial hardship. His father has insisted he sees his doctor.

Daniel's cue to consult with the doctor was his father's insistence. However, the underlying reason is that he is increasingly angry and upset, feeling sad and resentful, and his primary concern is that if this carries on, he might lose the job he got after he has studied so hard and long. He is displaying a range of emotional and behavioural symptoms which could signify a mental health disorder.

Clearly, there is not enough information here to determine whether Daniel's anger is a result of personality, pressure or pathology. However, this is a common presentation that could be any of the three. Let us imagine that Daniel is indeed suffering from depression, i.e. short circuit pathology; this would be a perfectly plausible presentation of such an illness. Daniel may have the insight to know this, and come to the doctor specifically with this preconception. However, it is equally possible that Daniel has assumed that his anger is a function of his personality or indeed of the pressure his life has put upon him.

Case study - Daniel

If Daniel had assumed that his personality was the problem, for example, he might come in and say:

'I'm just a worrier, doctor, and always have been; this is normal for me – I just get angry when I worry'

or

'I just get angry – it's just how my brain deals with things – other people do their thing, I get angry'

or

'I've been like this since school and university, I just need to change the way I am.'

Here, it can be seen that Daniel is pinning the blame for his outward symptom – the anger – on his personality make-up. He is saying he is an 'angry' person and always has been. There may or may not be some truth in this statement – ultimately we don't know yet. However, if he is suffering from a mental illness, the assumption of personality being the cause of anger is not correct. This would be an example of a mismatch between actual cause and assumed cause.

Case study - Daniel

Daniel may blame his life pressure for the anger. He may say:

'How can I not feel angry? Look at how I've been treated'

or

'How can I feel any different, given what's happened in my life?'

or

'I will no longer be angry when my boss sorts out the mess he has created!'

Here you can see that Daniel is saying that the anger is a direct and rational result of the life pressures and events he has gone through. Again, this is likely to be a factor. However, again, if there is an underlying pathology, in this case possible depression, he will be incorrectly assuming the anger is entirely driven by life events and the depression itself will be left undiagnosed.

These two mismatches of assumption vs. actual cause of a patient's symptoms are some of the biggest causes of untreated mental health conditions. This is where using the short circuit tool with patients can have its biggest impact.

Case study - Daniel

Daniel may arrive with a preconception of a mental health problem:

'I think I might be suffering from a mental illness and I would like some help with this'

or

'Things have changed – I'm not myself – I think I may have depression.'

Since personality, pressure and pathology could be driving Daniel's physical manifestations in a very similar way, it is easy to see how he could get the underlying cause confused. Any of the three Ps could be making him angry. The skill of the clinician, in partnership with the patient, will be to determine what the real underlying cause is and focus the treatment on that.

2.5.3 Comparing actual and assumed causes

Consider the table below, showing actual vs. assumed causes of a patient's emotional symptoms. However, before doing so, there are a few important points to consider.

First, it is important to remember, of course, that these separate boxes do not exist in isolation or with a distinct boundary. In reality, human patients present in a consultation with a complex and varied mixture of these boxes. They should be used to help determine the path the consultation can take and can be used as a reference point to understand why certain aspects of the diagnosis and treatment have succeeded or failed.

The second caveat is the definition of 'assumed' and 'actual'. In this illustration, I have defined the 'assumed' as the patient's pre-consultation impression. In other words, this is the thought process that the patient brings with them.

You also need to consider what the 'actual' means. There is no quick, simple test that you can do to define what the actual underlying source of the problem is. In this illustration, the 'actual' will, in reality, be the diagnostic conclusion of the consultation, or indeed series of consultations. This could, of course, be wrong. In further sections we will consider how you can use your skill and judgement to help determine where the 'actual' lies.

With that said, however, let's consider some of the scenarios clinicians commonly find in consultations, in the table below.

		ASSUMED		
		Personality	Pressure	Pathology
ACTUAL	Personality	The emotion is normal for their personality	Emotional state is a feature of personality but they blame life stressors	Emotional state is a feature of personality but they assume mental illness
	Pressure	Patients blame themselves but emotional state is a result of stress	Emotion is a result of life stressors and they recognise this	A mental illness is assumed but life stressors are the cause
	Pathology	**Mental illness**		
		These people blame themselves but have a treatable illness	Patients with a treatable illness who assume their state is due to life stressors	Patient correctly assumes that illness is present

Take the columns as being what the patient has assumed is the issue, and the rows as what the underlying issue may be. Of course in the first meeting with the patient you will not know the actual cause and may take some time to ascertain the assumed cause.

Taking each box from left to right and top to bottom, we see a number of scenarios.

ASSUMED: Personality

ACTUAL: Personality

They may be facing difficulties in life and have some emotional sequelae of that. The emotional state displayed will be normal for their own personality. There are many different human beings, each with a unique personality, and different people respond differently in various scenarios. This is normal. They correctly recognise that any issues could be dealt with using changes to lifestyle and attitudes – if this is what they desire. These people do not have a mental health issue and do not feel that they have. They are unlikely to present very often to the medical profession, nor are we especially concerned for their mental wellbeing. Those that actively seek to change themselves may find that they can mould their personality to a degree.

What if Daniel was here?:

Daniel's emotional and behavioural symptoms		Anger, irritability, resentfulness, outbursts	
What does Daniel think is the cause?	**What is the actual cause?**	**What does Daniel think will help?**	**What is likely to help?**
This is simply a feature of his underlying personality	This is his underlying personality	He may not wish to change anything but he would think that self-improvement strategies would be the answer. He would not have seen the doctor if it wasn't for his father	Self-help Personal coaching

ASSUMED: Pressure

ACTUAL: Personality

This is a difficult call to make. Here, the individual has assumed that the level of external stressor, or life pressure, is to blame for their demeanour and emotion. In actual fact, the stressor may not be all that great and their own personality make-up is the main factor. They may have some emotional sequelae but in fact, changing their life stressors might not, in this instance, make much difference to the emotional phenotype. They may present to the medical profession although they don't at heart feel they have a medical diagnosis. They may, however, ask for a sick note at times to relieve what they perceive to be work stress. It is possible that personality disorders exist in this group. People in this group may experience similar emotional responses in a wide variety of different situations.

What if Daniel was here?:

Daniel's emotional and behavioural symptoms		Anger, irritability, resentfulness, outbursts	
What does Daniel think is the cause?	**What is the actual cause?**	**What does Daniel think will help?**	**What is likely to help?**
He assumes the life pressure he is under is making him justifiably angry and irritable	This is his underlying personality	He wants a change to his circumstances in his workplace	Self-help Personal coaching

ASSUMED: Pathology

ACTUAL: Personality

This individual will consult with the doctor as they have assumed that a mental health diagnosis is at play. Naturally, there will be an expectation that the doctor will be able to help them with their issues. As above, since the medical diagnosis of a 'short circuit' pathology is not present, it is unlikely that medical therapies, including talking, behavioural or pharmacological, will work. Whilst it is outside the scope of this book, it is possible that some forms of personality disorder will exist. This patient will be a regular attendee and may suffer the disappointment of multiple treatment failures. A lifestyle-based approach may well be part of the answer, but care must be taken to ensure the patient's own assumptions are challenged and a consensus is reached.

What if Daniel was here?:

Daniel's emotional and behavioural symptoms		Anger, irritability, resentfulness, outbursts	
What does Daniel think is the cause?	**What is the actual cause?**	**What does Daniel think will help?**	**What is likely to help?**
He feels he has a mental health condition like depression	The emotional response is a feature of his underlying personality	He will see a medic and may assume that an antidepressant will work, but it is unlikely to	Self-help Personal coaching

ASSUMED: Personality

ACTUAL: Pressure

Many people live their lives in this state. Such individuals are under a great deal of stress but blame themselves. They may or may not present to the doctor but will often have a self-deprecating demeanour when they do. Their emotional response to the pressure they are under will often be very rational, but they will not recognise the stressor; moreover, they will assume that other people are able to cope but they themselves are not. The person needs the emotional support of the medical professional and must be reassured that their feelings toward their stressors are common, but they do not have a mental health diagnosis. Social prescribing may be of value (see *Section 6.3.3*).

What if Daniel was here?:

Daniel's emotional and behavioural symptoms		Anger, irritability, resentfulness, outbursts	
What does Daniel think is the cause?	**What is the actual cause?**	**What does Daniel think will help?**	**What is likely to help?**
This is simply a feature of his underlying personality	His emotional and physical response is entirely natural and rational in the face of the high level of life stress	He will be blaming himself and feeling that he has let himself down and will be trying self-help improvement strategies	Reduction of stress levels Some time off work Social prescribing

ASSUMED: Pressure

ACTUAL: Pressure

Here, the individual has correctly assumed that the level of external stressor, or life pressure, is to blame for their demeanour. There is often a very rational state of emotion associated with the stressor, whether that be sadness as part of grief or worry about job insecurity. They are not displaying signs of pathology (as described in *Sections 4.2.5 and 4.2.6*) and instinctively do not believe they are ill – just overburdened with stress. If they do present to the doctor it will often be to help them with the pressure, such as asking for a sick note. Social prescribing may be of value.

What if Daniel was here?:

Daniel's emotional and behavioural symptoms	Anger, irritability, resentfulness, outbursts		
What does Daniel think is the cause?	**What is the actual cause?**	**What does Daniel think will help?**	**What is likely to help?**
The level of life stress	The level of life stress	Reduction of life stressors	Reduction of stress levels
			Some time off work
			Social prescribing

ASSUMED: Pathology

ACTUAL: Pressure

This is a scenario that many doctors find themselves in. The patient has assumed that their state is a result of pathology but in fact their problems lie almost entirely within the fact that their life stressors are far too great. Interventions for depression are unlikely to make much difference and the patient may well keep returning, unimproved, following treatments. Doctors of these patients may attempt to influence the patient's life stressors and in some cases can find success in this, whilst at other times such attempts may meet with limited success. Social prescribing may have a part to play in helping these people, as the solution will require a change to circumstance rather than treatment of a pathology.

What if Daniel was here?:

Daniel's emotional and behavioural symptoms		Anger, irritability, resentfulness, outbursts	
What does Daniel think is the cause?	**What is the actual cause?**	**What does Daniel think will help?**	**What is likely to help?**
A mental health disorder such as depression or anxiety	The level of life stress	A medical treatment such as an SSRI	Reduction of stress levels Some time off work Social prescribing

The last row is where there is indeed a mental health diagnosis – the short circuit exists. Here is where the short circuit tool can be extremely helpful in helping you navigate through the consultation and help change the patient's view of the cause of their distress.

ASSUMED: Personality

ACTUAL: Pathology

This common scenario is where the short circuit comes into its own. This is a person who is suffering from a condition such as depression or anxiety. They have often suffered for a very long time. They will have assumed that this is a natural part of their personality. An example would be a man who has a generalised anxiety disorder but has simply put himself down as a worrier all his life. In this scenario, where the doctor can see signs of mental illness (such as those described in *Chapter 4*), but the patient simply doesn't believe it is, this book and the short circuit tool can be of great value. Treatments will have a good chance of success.

What if Daniel was here?:

Daniel's emotional and behavioural symptoms		Anger, irritability, resentfulness, outbursts	
What does Daniel think is the cause?	**What is the actual cause?**	**What does Daniel think will help?**	**What is likely to help?**
That this is simply a function of his personality	He has a treatable mental illness	Improving himself 'Getting his head together'	A recognised treatment for a mental health disorder such as CBT or an SSRI

ASSUMED: Pressure

ACTUAL: Pathology

This is another very common scenario. This patient is suffering from a mental health condition but has assumed the problem is the life stressor. They may have suffered for a long time or not, depending on the timescale of the stressor. They will have assumed that their feelings and symptoms are a simple response to the life stressor. A bereaved widow, for example, may develop depression and feel the only solution would be to bring back her late husband. Again, the simple short circuit tool can be used to explain to the patient that their pathology can be treated despite the persistence of their pressures. These patients can become very ill as they have an underlying pathology alongside a real pressure. Their short circuit will be persistently buzzing and it is fundamentally important to help them realise there is a very treatable component. Treatments have a very good chance of success and the successful treatment of these patients, as well as in the category above, is incredibly rewarding to the doctor, and the relief afforded to the patient – who initially felt helpless – is immeasurable.

What if Daniel was here?:

Daniel's emotional and behavioural symptoms		Anger, irritability, resentfulness, outbursts	
What does Daniel think is the cause?	**What is the actual cause?**	**What does Daniel think will help?**	**What is likely to help?**
That his life stressors are the reason he is angry	He has a treatable mental illness	Changing his life stressors such as his boss	A recognised treatment for a mental health disorder such as CBT or an SSRI

ASSUMED: Pathology

ACTUAL: Pathology

There are many patients who do recognise pathology when it is actually there in terms of mental illness. This may be due to a good background understanding or it may be because they have suffered in the past and recognise the symptoms. Again, because the underlying problems include pathology, the treatments have a good chance of success. Care must still be taken, however, as even where patients are very open to the possibility of illness, there may still be difficulty in understanding the connection between mental and physical symptoms. If stigma did not exist for mental illness and if mental illness was more 'visible', I feel that many more people who actually suffer pathology would fall into this category, rather than assuming their problems were related to their personality or pressure.

What if Daniel was here?:

Daniel's emotional and behavioural symptoms		Anger, irritability, resentfulness, outbursts	
What does Daniel think is the cause?	What is the actual cause?	What does Daniel think will help?	What is likely to help?
That he is suffering from a condition like depression	He has a treatable mental illness	Some medical intervention for his mental health	A recognised treatment for a mental health disorder such as CBT or an SSRI

The matrix described above gives nine separate scenarios, each of which will give the consulter a different challenge. In the real world, patients do not fall neatly into exactly one box but many doctors will recognise consultations like each of those described above.

Clearly the short circuit tool is best placed to deal with those patients where there is a pathology present, but for any number of the reasons already discussed, the patient does not believe in it. I personally feel that this third row – where there is pathology with or without the patient realising it – is where there is the most urgent need of the medical profession's attention. This is where the undiagnosed pathology sits – this is where there are ill patients who have been blinded to that fact by the stigma of the society they live in.

Chapter 3

The short circuit as a tool: a practical approach

3.1 Mental health presentations

> **What you'll learn in this section**
> Mental health disorders present in a number of ways and the consultation can be influenced by stigma. The short circuit tool can be introduced to the consultation at a number of points to help with this.
>
> **How this helps**
> You can now see where the short circuit tool fits within the consultation.

Mental health illness can present itself in your clinic in a number of different ways. Amongst these would be that the patient:

- presents with typical emotional symptoms of mental illness
- presents with typical physical symptoms of mental illness
- is encouraged by others to see the doctor
- already has a mental health diagnosis and is re-presenting after a change or relapse of symptoms
- presents after scoring high on a screening tool
- presents with a completely different medical problem and a mental health condition is suspected by the clinician.

This list is not exhaustive but with every one of these presentations, there may be an element of stigma, preconception and misconception, and this has the potential of adversely guiding the consultation and resulting in a suboptimal outcome for the patient.

Whilst it is not the intention of this book to guide you through a full mental health history and examination, it is here to help reduce or eliminate the stigma and misconception so that the right diagnosis and management plan can be arrived at safely and quickly. Ultimately this should help the patient get better sooner and should help the clinician in their consultation and any future encounters with the patient.

Consider this pathway, which is a fairly typical, if a little simplified, journey of a consultation:

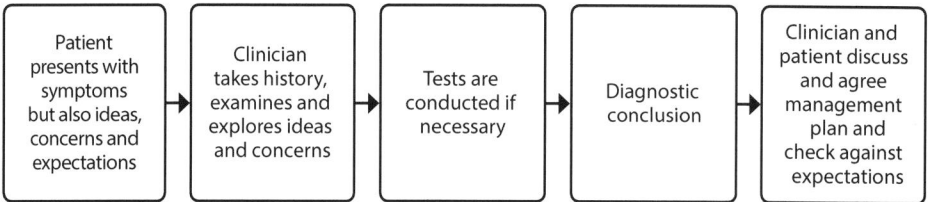

This will be familiar to clinicians across many specialities and forms the taught method for medical students, doctors and nurses. Using the headings above, almost any medical illness can be broken down, for teaching and training purposes, into its symptoms, examination signs, tests, diagnostic criteria and management. Indeed, medical textbooks will often do this.

Mental illness is no different, in that at its core it has a set of symptoms and signs, diagnostic methods and a well-evidenced suite of treatment options. In *Chapter 4: Mental illnesses in detail* these are discussed and considered in more detail for the common primary care mental health presentations.

The added complication with mental health diagnosis is the very high levels of stigma, preconception and misconception that exist. These are present in many other forms of illness and disability but they are very much more prevalent for mental illness.

The short circuit tool helps you with these added challenges in the mental health consultation. Once you have used the tool to overcome these hurdles, you will be in a good position to offer the patient interventions and treatments for their condition in the normal way.

Consider this diagram which suggests where the tool would sit in the consultation process.

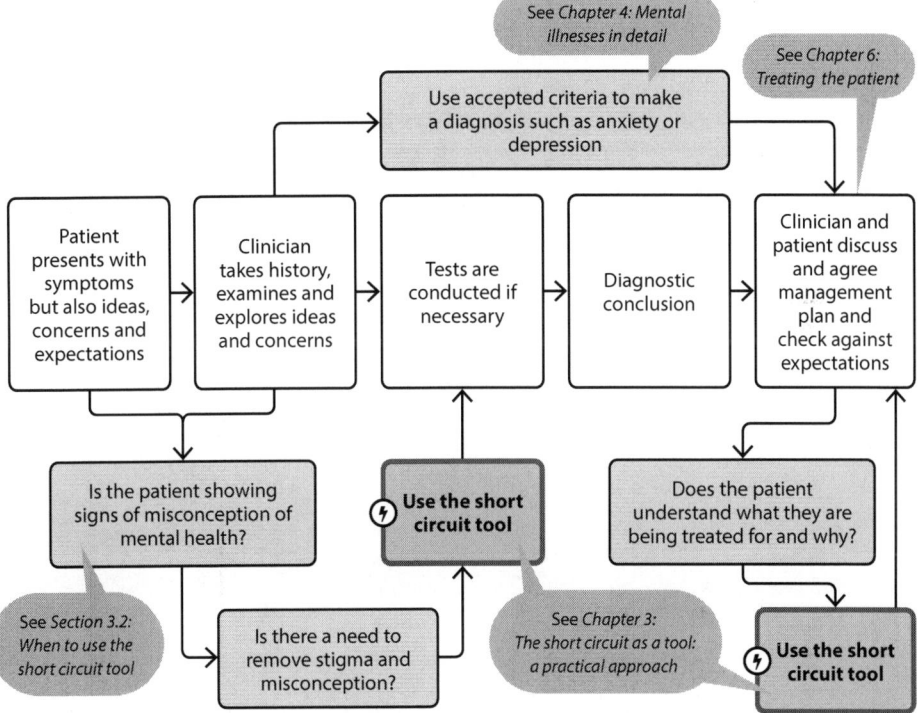

The baseline process of making a mental health diagnosis hasn't changed. The short circuit does not make a diagnosis, nor does it form a treatment plan. What it does is to fundamentally help with the added complication of patient understanding associated with this type of illness.

Section 3.2: When to use the short circuit tool will help with identifying the need to start using the tool. *Section 3.3: Using the short circuit tool in a consultation* will show you how to deliver the message in a short time.

In *Chapter 4: Mental illnesses in detail* you will get a detailed breakdown of the important signs and symptoms of each of the main clinical diagnoses seen in primary care. *Chapter 5* then provides details of common physical illnesses which have a mental health component. *Chapter 6* will help you master the treatment options at your disposal.

3.2 When to use the short circuit tool

What you'll learn in this section
How to look for the presentation cues from the patient and the different types of cues which can present themselves.

How this helps
The short circuit tool is a quick and easy way to help patients understand mental health better, but you need to know when to start using it for maximum impact. By looking for these cues, you will be able to bring it out at the right moments for the right patients.

Mental health diagnoses can arise from a number of different starting scenarios. Sometimes the patient will arrive with a clear impression of the underlying cause of their illness:

Patient

'Doctor, I think I have depression.'

Other times the presentation is of a gamut of emotional symptoms:

'I am feeling down and hopeless'
'I continuously worry'
'I am struggling emotionally'

Mental illness also has numerous well-recognised physical symptoms and this may be the primary presentation:

'I can't sleep'
'I feel short of breath and have palpitations'
'I feel bloated and get intermittent abdominal pain'

Physical symptoms will have a range of possible differential diagnoses and it is, of course, important to be satisfied that other causes have been ruled out. For example, shortness of breath can be associated with asthma as well as anxiety, and palpitations have numerous cardiac and pharmacological causes as well as anxiety.

The use of the short circuit tool comes when there is a likelihood that a mental health diagnosis is at play. The possibility of such a diagnosis may come very early on in the consultation, or may come after a number of separate consultations. It becomes exceedingly powerful when misconception or stigma is picked up in the consultation. Using the three Ps concept, when stigma is present, pathology is missed and the effects of pathology are assumed to be the result of a personal character trait or the presence of life stressors.

3.2.1 Scenarios where the tool could be used

Over the past 6 or 7 years as a GP since I've been using the short circuit tool I've found many useful scenarios where it has had a huge benefit to both the patient and me as the clinician. However, there are a number of specific scenarios where the use of the tool is extremely helpful. These are some of those scenarios.

Using the assumed vs. actual table from *Section 2.5.3*, there are two scenarios where pathology may be present but incorrectly attributed to something else.

1. Pathology confused with personality
2. Pathology confused with pressure.

A third scenario exists which, although not unique to mental health conditions, is more pronounced in this field; that is the perceived mismatch of physical symptoms to underlying diagnosis. Mental illness causes physical symptoms. However, this connection is not always obvious to the population generally. It is natural for any patient to consider possible causes for their symptoms before they enter a consultation. When the connection is not obvious there can be confusion and resistance, and this scenario is considered at the end of this chapter. For example, patients who present with palpitations may be resistant, for a number of reasons, to considering anxiety as the cause over a cardiac problem.

Pathology confused with personality

In this scenario, the patient has a belief that illness such as anxiety or depression is a function of the personality. Take the following patient:

Case study - Sandra

Sandra is an advertising executive who has presented with contact dermatitis on her palms several times over the last few consultations. She has been given steroids and emollients. You find that she is using alcohol hand sanitiser numerous times over the course of the day. On questioning, it is actually up to 50 times in a day. She works in an office environment and often from home and there is nothing unusual about her life routines. She has two school-age children who she drops off in the morning. Her husband picks them up. She does her weekly shopping and often feels unclean if she has entered a high street shop for anything from clothes to groceries. She feels that without using the hand sanitiser she is dirty and at risk of infectious disease and can often feel uncomfortable and vulnerable without its use. This fear of being unclean can be a persistent and intrusive thought.

The above example may suggest to the clinician that Sandra has a degree of OCD. However, Sandra may not see it this way. She may, as many of the population do, have a concept of what OCD is. However, she may not see that this is something that affects her. She may well consider the repeated hand washing as simply a feature of her diligent and risk-averse personality. Here, a possible mental illness is being confused with a personality trait. With this misconception in mind, Sandra may not have considered OCD as a diagnosis for one of the following two reasons:

a) *'My personality is not compatible with mental illness'* or *'I'm not the sort of person who gets mental illness'*
b) *'This is just a normal feature of my personality, not a mental illness.'*

Mental illness is not compatible with my personality

When the patient has a misconceived link between mental illness and personality, they may be at pains to state that they could not have such a condition, as their personality is not compatible with this.

Case study – Sandra

Sandra may say:

'I am a very experienced executive, I lead a big team and I am successful, I therefore don't have OCD.'

'I am not the sort of person that panics or worries, OCD is something that only people like that have.'

'How could I have OCD? Look at what I have achieved and how strong I have to be to do my job.'

'I'm not that type of person.'

> Many people can feel genuinely offended by the suggestion that a mental health disorder could be present. The diagnosis of an illness may be seen as an affront to their person and their sense of self.

As you can see from these statements, Sandra is assuming that a mental health problem is a function of personality. Sandra has already given some background about herself and her life which may give you some insight into her personality. Here, she has incorrectly assumed that because of these personality traits, she can't have a mental health disorder.

Many people have this misconception. When this is present, such people can feel genuinely offended by the suggestion that a mental health disorder could be present. The diagnosis of an illness may be seen as an affront to their person and their sense of self. For this reason they may not wish to entertain the idea. This form of stigma comes from the incorrect belief that only certain types of people get mental illness. Often the stereotypes of this 'type of person' will have negative associations attached to them – such as weakness, laziness and ineptitude. Therefore giving a patient such a diagnosis may be received as if they are being told that they have a defective personality of some description.

An important part of the effective management of patients in this situation is to help them separate their own notion of their own personality with a mental health disorder. Sandra is a proud, independent, strong and successful individual. There is no need for her to feel that this is in any way changed or challenged by the fact that she may have a mental health diagnosis.

Clinicians will often find themselves in this scenario and it is a clear indication to start the use of the short circuit tool.

Consultation tip

Sometimes giving a few examples of famous personalities who have suffered with a mental health disorder can dispel the myth that weakness of person or their mental constitution is a feature of mental illness.

Talk about Winston Churchill. This is a character from British and world history who is hardly associated with any weakness of personality. He suffered with very significant depression.

Talk about Andrew "Freddie" Flintoff. Freddie, being an international sporting hero, is hardly associated with weakness. Yet he suffered very significant depression. Many of the world's top Olympic athletes will take time out to help their mental health.

Mention Albert Einstein. Albert Einstein is synonymous with the notion of genius; hardly a man of weak mind. Yet he suffered very significant depression causing angry outbursts and significant personal dishevelment.

Refer to Adele, one of the world's best-selling music artists and an icon of her generation; she has spoken publicly about the significant anxiety she suffers.

Mention Virginia Woolf, the colossus of English literature, who suffered severe depression.

These examples should help dispel the notion in your patient that there is a connection between weakness of mind, body or personality and mental health disorders such as depression or anxiety.

This is my personality, not a mental illness

This is another 'mix-up' between personality and pathology; however, this has significantly different implications.

Here, the patient has assumed that the traits that they are exhibiting are simply a feature of their underlying personality, when in reality they are suffering from a treatable illness.

Case study - Sandra

Sandra may come in and say:

'No, this isn't OCD, it's just how I have always been.'
'I thought it was normal to be this concerned about hygiene.'
'Washing is just my personal mechanism for coping with life pressure.'
'Surely this is just something that everybody does?'

These statements effectively normalise an illness by making the sufferer believe that their personality is simply one that requires them to behave in a certain way. Often these people have lived with a treatable mental health disorder for many years and will sometimes have built up strategies to manage the disorder – sometimes very successfully and other times not. Illnesses such as anxiety, depression and OCD are present in people who may not have much concept that they are even there.

A common example is a generalised anxiety disorder or a social anxiety disorder. These illnesses, if they appear in a teenager, may lead them to believe that they are just the sort of person that is unable to be around others. This can have a severely deleterious effect on their life, social interaction and life chances such as career opportunities. After a period of time they simply believe that this is normal for them. Rather than seek help, they simply adjust what they do to make the symptoms of their illness as less pronounced as possible.

Whereas in the previous scenario the patient may be resistant to a diagnosis because of the feeling that it suggested that their personality is at fault, here the reverse may be true. The patient assumes that their personality is one that simply suffers from a range of difficulties and actually they may be open to the possibility that pathological process may be involved. For some people in this scenario, the notion that they may find some relief with active treatment can be a great source of hope and inspiration.

This is another clear-cut scenario for starting the use of the short circuit tool.

Pathology confused with pressure

Here we have another incorrect assumption. As with the previous example, there are two opposite scenarios. There is an incorrect belief that mental illness can only be associated with a certain degree of life pressure. Of course it's well recognised that life pressure can be a contributing factor to the start of mental illness. However, stresses can exist with or without mental illness and vice versa. Take the following patient example.

Case study - Ali

Ali is a 46-year-old bus driver who has been under significant financial strain for the last few years. He lives with his wife and three children and is concerned for the future of his own job. He feels that he has been the subject of bullying at work. Ali is significantly overweight and has recently had a diagnosis of type 2 diabetes. He has been started on metformin. His weight has been a significant source of embarrassment for him and despite efforts to get it down he has struggled. Ali has two older brothers and a younger sister. His older brother recently lost his 9-year-old son after battling acute lymphoblastic leukaemia. Over the last six months Ali has found it difficult to sleep and to concentrate, he has had increasing irritability resulting in arguments at work and home, and has noticed a decrease in his libido.

In this history you can see that Ali is showing some physical and emotional signs of depression although there are, of course, other possible diagnoses to explain his symptoms. A more in-depth analysis of depression is covered in *Section 4.2: Focus on depression*. Pathology, i.e. depression, could be at play. Let's consider how a confusion between pathology and pressure, using the three Ps model, could present itself. As with the confusion between pathology and personality, this particular situation has two modes:

> Illnesses such as anxiety, depression and OCD are present in people who may not have much concept that they are even there.

a) *The belief that pressure is the cause of symptoms, not pathology*
b) *The belief that pathology cannot be present without the relevant pressure.*

Pressure is the cause, not pathology

This may be suspected when the patient has a clear perception that the sum of their life pressures are the cause of their gamut of emotional symptoms. In this case take Ali's symptoms: difficulty in sleeping, difficulty in concentrating, irritability and argumentativeness, and loss of libido. Ali may have been encouraged to come to the doctor by his family or work colleagues. He may have come for some support with time off work.

> ### Case study - Ali
>
> If Ali was of the belief that his life pressures were the sole cause of these symptoms, he may come and say:
>
> *'Money is tight, my work and bosses are stressful, and these are the cause of my symptoms.'*
>
> *'It's very clear that anyone who had this boss would have the same set of symptoms as me.'*
>
> *'If only I could sort my money situation out, all of these symptoms would go away.'*
>
> *'You know what happened to my nephew – that is why I have these symptoms.'*

You can clearly see here that Ali is attributing the set of symptoms that he is displaying to his life pressures – predominantly his money situation, his torturous work situation and his family grief. Clearly these are significant stresses in his life and will surely be contributing to his emotional state. Obviously there is a degree of rationality around his demeanour. One would expect an element of worry associated with a potential loss of money, through loss of his job. One would associate a degree of anger with unfairness at work. The grief he is going through or has gone through is a natural response to his horrendous family bereavement. However, pathology may also be at play. We know that depression can occur in those who have very significant life stresses and those who do not. We also know that depression can be absent in those with significant life stresses.

If Ali is suffering from the pathology of depression, then he has incorrectly guessed that the cause of his symptoms is his life pressures. This is an example of confusion between pressure and pathology. It is fairly obvious why people generally would have this confusion. The gamut of emotional symptoms that occur with life pressures can mimic the gamut of symptoms that occur with depression. The pathology will of course be responsive to medical therapies and interventions; however, life pressures will not be affected by such.

In this scenario the clinician can use the short circuit tool to explain the difference between pressure and pathology.

Pathology cannot be present without pressure

The second type of confusion between pressure and pathology can come when there is an incorrect belief that a condition like depression cannot be present without the appropriate life stresses. There are a number of ways that this misconception can present in a consultation.

> ## Case study - Ali
>
> If Ali was of this belief he may say:
>
> *'I'm not depressed. I have some stress in my life but it's not enough to cause depression.'*
>
> *'My brother has lost his son. He's coping so there's no reason I should have depression.'*
>
> *'I have nothing to be depressed about. There are many more people in the world worse off than me.'*
>
> Or Ali may have heard from others:
>
> *'Pull yourself together, there are those in this world much worse off than you.'*

Here you can see the reverse problem. It is a common misconception that mental illness can only possibly be present with certain life stressors. This belief can cause a number of problems. First, people can live with the pain of guilt that they have a set of symptoms that they do not understand or do not believe they should have. Often people can compare themselves to others and find that because their set of stressors is not as bad, they should not suffer mental illness. This stigmatising belief can be perpetuated by others around them too.

It is a common misconception that mental illness can only possibly be present with certain life stressors.

Your task as a clinician here is to convey how the pathology of a mental illness is related to, but fundamentally separate from, the notion of life stresses. Again this is an ideal opportunity to start the short circuit tool in your consultation.

> ### Consultation tip
>
> When trying to dispel the connection between life pressure and mental illness, try saying this to patients – in relation to a condition such as depression:
>
> *'If it were the case that only people with severe life pressure have depression and only severe life pressure can cause depression, then we would see a very different pattern of illness across the country and across the globe. For example, all those that live in the slums of India or Brazil who ostensibly live difficult and stressful lives, should all suffer with depression. Equally those who live comfortable, financially stable and generally pleasant lives should not ever suffer with depression. In reality such an association does not exist.'*
>
> Most people can relate to this. They can clearly see that even people with lives more comfortable than theirs can suffer with depression. And they can clearly see that depression does not affect all people who live in much more difficult situations.
>
> This can help separate pathology and pressure.

Mental health pathology mixed up with physical health pathology

This is where the patient has a set of physical symptoms which they do not believe could be caused by a mental health disorder. It is natural for patients to come into a consultation with a concept of what might be wrong. It is almost unheard of, in the last 10 years, for people not to Google their symptoms. In fact, most of the medical profession encourages the use of patient self-help portals before seeking help from the NHS.

When a set of symptoms does not match with the patient's understanding of the possible differential diagnosis, it is easily possible to alienate the patient and it is important to carefully consider how this misunderstanding is rectified.

For example, palpitations can be caused by a number of conditions. Amongst others, these can include a primary cardiac dysfunction, hyperthyroidism or anxiety.

Consider Peter, our next patient case study:

Case study - Peter

Peter is a 19-year-old second-year university student studying sociology. He struggled in his first year but managed to get through. Over the last 9 months he's developed intermittent palpitations. These can be extremely distressing and can sometimes be associated with a feeling of shortness of breath. He says that these occur mainly in the evenings and are often short-lived but he can get many episodes over the course of the day. Peter's grandfather recently had an MI and now has heart failure. Peter has two cousins who have been treated for overactive thyroid glands. These symptoms have made Peter extremely worried, to the extent that it's affecting his university work. He also says that he has found it increasingly difficult to socialise because of the worry of the symptoms recurring.

Peter is clearly suffering from a set of distressing symptoms. He may have a number of ideas and concerns in the consulting room about what might be going on. Of course you will explore this with him. Clearly from the description given there is not enough information to make a diagnosis, but a number of things will be on your differential at this point. These could be palpitations due to a heart arrhythmia or an endocrine disorder, or they could be as a result of a panic disorder. You will need to investigate appropriately. Peter may find it difficult to consider anything other than the cardiac cause.

The resistance to entertaining the idea of a mental health cause of the palpitations may come from a lack of understanding of the connection but also there may be worry that the doctor is 'dismissing' the symptoms as 'just anxiety'. Equally there could be concern that the doctor may 'miss' a serious cardiac problem by being drawn too far into the mental health possibility.

> **Case study - Peter**
>
> Peter may say:
>
> *'I have a strong family history of cardiac problems and therefore this must be what's going on.'*
>
> *'I don't feel stressed when these come on – it can't be "anxiety".'*
>
> *'I understand anxiety can make you worry, but I have real symptoms – I'm not making these up.'*
>
> *'How can anxiety cause heart palpitations? It must be a heart problem.'*
>
> These are all sensible, intelligent and rational questions and comments.

The basic premise in Peter's mind here is that anxiety is a different thing to the physical health symptoms he is describing and experiencing. The clinician's job is to carefully explain how a mental health disorder can in fact be the cause of his symptoms. Peter may also have the same misconceptions about personality and pressure but here there is also the specific confusion that a mental health pathology can't be the cause of a physical set of symptoms.

In *Section 5.1.2: Another mechanism for somatic symptoms*, there is a more in-depth analysis of how mental health disorders cause physical symptoms and how you can help your patients understand this.

This presentation is a good cue to start the short circuit tool.

3.3 Using the short circuit tool in a consultation

> **What you'll learn in this section**
> This is a practical guide to using the tool in a patient consultation.
>
> **How this helps**
> This will help you use the tool effectively in a short time and with practice you will be able to do this in minutes.

Once you have made the decision to use the short circuit tool, it's time to explain this to the patient. This needs to be quick and impactful. After all, many of you, certainly at the time of writing, will have a ten-minute consultation. You will be helping the patient to visualise mental illness and remove the stigma associated with it. As such, your explanation to the patient will need to be visual too.

I have been using this technique for at least six years now, and have honed it down to a few minutes. With practice, this is not difficult to achieve.

Before you embark on this, the consultation will have had some clues that the underlying diagnosis is within the mental health sphere. You will have suggested this to the patient and you will have picked up some reaction from the patient, who may feel stigmatised by such a diagnosis. The previous chapter gives some common scenarios when this may occur, but these examples are by no means exhaustive. I have used this tool with patients who have been treated for depression or anxiety for many years and found that it helped them.

Be aware also, that at this stage you may not have made a definitive diagnosis, you are simply enabling an open-minded exploration. You are not necessarily suggesting that the patient has pathology, but allowing them to see mental health pathology as a possible and credible differential diagnosis.

There are a few ways you can do this visually in your consultation:

- Draw out the diagrams in front of the patient
- Use the templates on the Resources tab at **www.scionpublishing.com/shortcircuit** to go through with your patient on the screen.
  - There are two versions of the templates, one with some annotated comments and one without – you may find one better for your consultation and the other better for patients to see themselves.

This tutorial is given for drawing with the patient. It may save you some time to use a pre-printed version from the website above. If you do download the pre-printed version or use the webpages as your guide, you can still follow the tutorial for its explanations to the patient through the steps.

Step 1: Setting the scene

Explain to the patient what you are going to do. Tell them that you are going to try to present mental health in a way they may not have seen before. Say how, once you have shown them a new way of looking at it, it will help them 'see' depression or anxiety in the same way as they 'see' any other physical health illness. Also say how this will help them separate themselves as an individual from illness, and how illness is a different thing to the stresses they are facing in their life.

> **Key concepts**
>
> - *'I'm going to **show you a new way** of looking at mental illness*
> - *You will be able to **"see" the illness** that is often called "invisible"*
> - *You will be able to **separate out your own personality** from the illness and you will see how the illness is different to your life stressors.'*

Step 2: Describing normal life and its problems

If you are drawing this out in front of the patient, you will now need a piece of paper. In my consulting room, we have slips of paper which we give out to patients to instruct reception to book follow-up appointments, blood tests, nurse reviews and such-like. These are about a half to a third of an A4 sheet and provide the perfect size. Any smaller might look scrappy and difficult to follow.

Start your drawing with a cloud-like bubble, which you explain to your patient is your depiction of a brain. This is usually followed by an apology, on my part, for being a dreadful artist! After six years, my circles still look like those of a primary school child!

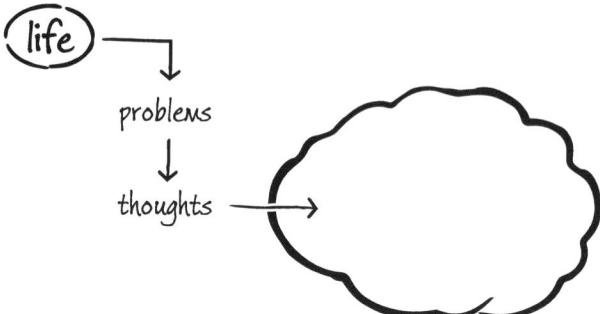

On the page, write LIFE at the top and explain that there are an almost infinite variety of different lives being lived. Of the 7.5 billion humans living on the planet today, no two are the same. This should all be very rudimentary and self-explanatory.

Under this, you draw an arrow from LIFE and write 'problems'. You will now explain to the patient that different lives have different problems. And with an almost infinite number of lives, there are an almost infinite number of different possible problems. These can include money, family, relationships, work, housing, etc. At this stage, you might wish to relate to some of the patient's individual life problems that you may know about at this point in the consultation. It is very important at this stage to express to the patient that these life problems are not the mental health illness.

Finally, under problems, you write 'thoughts'. Explain to the patient that what you mean by this is all of the active conscious thoughts that appear in anyone's head as a result of the problems that appear in their lives. These thoughts can take any number of different forms, characters and qualities. They could be thoughts about past events, thoughts about what happened earlier today or thoughts about things that haven't even happened yet. The thoughts could be big, small, dark, rational, zany, trivial, horrific – or indeed anything. Explain to the patient that because all our lives have some degree of problem issues, we all have thoughts that pop up all of the time. Make sure you get across that this is all normal. Again, it is vitally important to get across that the thoughts themselves, their existence or their nature, are not a mental illness.

Key concepts

- The patient's **life is unique**
- Their life, along with billions of other lives in the world, **has problems inherent** to it – however, the problems themselves are not mental illness
- The **problems give people thoughts**; many different and varied thoughts. Even when the thoughts are dark or feel irrational, they do not represent the mental illness – they are present in all people.

It is vitally important to get across to the patient that the thoughts themselves, their existence or their nature, are not a mental illness.

Step 3: Describing normal thought process

You will now start to show the patient how these thoughts are carried through their brain. At this juncture, if you haven't already, it's important to get across that what you are about to tell them is not a formal, physically accurate or anatomically literal description of what happens. This is a metaphor for the passage of thought. There is obviously not an A, B, C or D in the mind as separate lobar parts of the brain, nor do thoughts move in a simple four-step process. The A–B–C–D 'train of thought' is here specifically to illustrate that thoughts progress through the mind, reaching some end-point.

Take your drawing and now insert an arrow from the 'thoughts', going into the brain at point A. Continue this with arrows that follow the process through the brain, through B to D, finally departing. The departure from the active mind will be at one of two end-points. The thought may be 'solved' or it may be 'stored'.

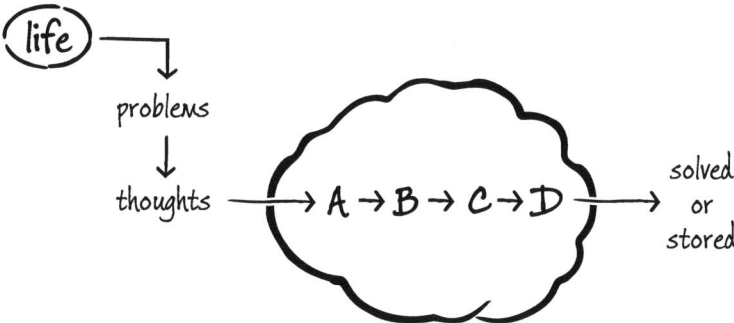

It may be useful to give an example of a thought process that could end in each of these eventualities. For example, the thought could be related to a financial problem. If a bill that needs to be paid is in the current train of thought, it may progress through a number of phases. Once the solution to the money shortage is found, the thought is considered 'solved'. On the other hand, consider a thought about a loved one who died some time ago. It could be about a memory or loss or about missing the individual. Of course, the person is not going to come back, so it can't be 'solved'; however, there is a mechanism for this to be stored, in a memory, so that it no longer occupies the active mind. This stored thought may come back into the active mind at another point in the future, maybe the next day, perhaps not for another week or month. But it no longer occupies the current flow of thought.

I would reiterate at this point that you have not described anything which could be called a mental illness, state again that any number of irrational or odd-sounding thoughts appear in the minds of all people, but the fact that they progress to some endpoint makes these a normal passage of thought.

Key concepts

- **All people have thoughts** relating to the problems in their lives.
- The thoughts can induce sadness, worry, anger or any number of emotions, but **the nature and character of the thoughts do not represent mental illness**.
- Thoughts will progress through the mind **and reach some endpoint** – either solved or stored – in a sort of 'mental workflow'.

Step 4: Describing stress and life pressure

At points in the patient's life they will have an abundance of life problems, pressures and stressors. In times like this, the problems generating thoughts will be higher and the number of different thoughts entering the brain will be greater. This means that the 'traffic' flowing through will be greater too.

You can represent this on your drawing with extra arrows going through the machinery.

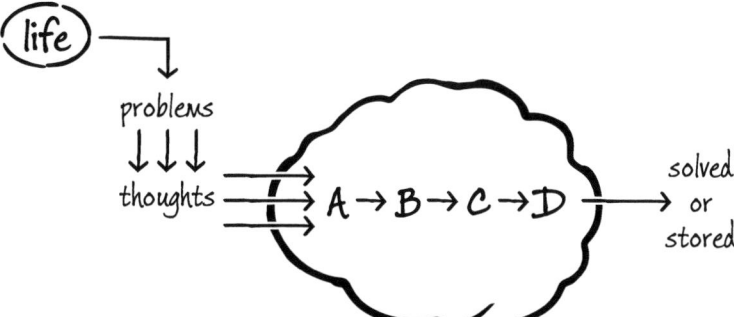

This will have its impact on the individual – we can call this 'stress'. Their mind is having to do more, and dealing with a greater over-all workload will be tiring for the brain, just as would be the case for any other organ of the body.

The important thing to convey to the patient here is that this is, again, all normal, and does not represent a mental illness.

Key concepts

- At time of **stress** the **workflow or 'traffic'** through the mind is greater.
- The greater quantity of thoughts during this time will induce emotion and will tire the mind – just like any other organ of the body.
- Despite this, the stressed state is not mental illness. Thoughts will progress through the mind **and reach some end-point** – either solved or stored. There are just a very large number of them!

Step 5: Visualising the mental illness - the short circuit

Tell the patient you are now about to show them the effect of what a mental illness is. You will now draw the short circuit loop between C and B.

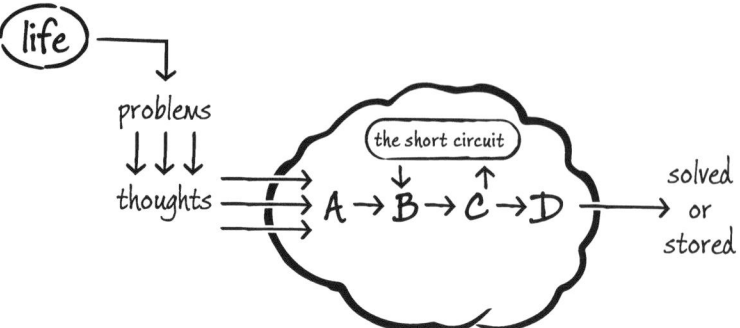

You can now describe any thought process, starting with a life problem entering the mind at the beginning, point A. It now tries to get through to some logical end-point where it is either solved or stored, but after C, instead of moving to D, it bounces back to B. It now cycles, almost constantly, between B and C – back and forth, back and forth. In this case the thought is trapped by the short circuit and can neither be solved nor stored. Follow this up with another addition to the diagram:

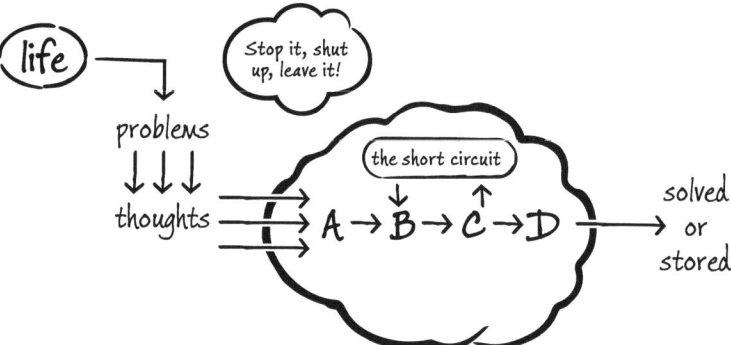

I draw this 'back of the brain' thought bubble onto the diagram to give it a visual presence. For every patient I have ever shown this to, it has been fairly obvious that this is, again, not a literal, anatomically or physiologically correct depiction of the organ of the brain. Nevertheless, I still point this out!

This 'back of the brain' is trying to tell the mind to 'stop it'. It is saying 'shut up,' 'stop overthinking it,' 'move on'.

You now have a picture in front of you that you can point at with the patient. The mental illness is the loop back, and the battle with the 'back of the brain'. The problem thoughts are now trapped, bouncing back and forth. Show your patient the loop and explain that this is the health disorder. Show your patient that this can exist with or without certain life problems. You can physically point to the two different parts of the diagram that represent life problems and mental illness as two separate things – one may be influencing the other but they are separate parts of the thinking process. Show them that the loop can appear, as an illness, in a person of any sort, just like cancer.

Show them, perhaps with a little line through the short circuit, that once the loop is broken, they will feel relief from their symptoms, even though the stresses and strains of their life may still be present. This is fundamentally important as it will set out what you as the physician can help hugely with. It will help guide your current consultation and future consultations.

> Once the loop is broken, the patient will feel relief from their symptoms, even though the stresses and strains of their life may still be present.

> **Key concepts**
>
> - You have now **'visualised' the mental illness** for the patient.
> - You have shown them that the life problems and thoughts that they are bound to create are in fact a slightly separate thing to the mental illness.
> - You have shown them the part that can be fixed.

Step 5: Give the patient a chance to reflect

It is now important to stop. Take a breath and consolidate what you have just shown your patient with their experience and understanding. Ask the question:

'Does what I have just described feel familiar to you?'

As I have stated previously, this tool should not be used in isolation to make a diagnosis of depression, anxiety or any other mental illness. It does not have the evidence base to do that. However, since this thought bouncing is such a strong feature of these disorders, you may want to reflect on your patient's answer. If the description you have just given, and the drawing you have just made, result in an expression of immediate understanding from your patient then I feel this can help lend evidence to the diagnosis of a condition such as anxiety or depression. However, if the patient feels no familiarity with what you have just described, then it may refute such an idea.

> ### Key concepts
>
> - **Stop and reflect** – does this all sound to the patient like a good description of what is going on in their head?
> - **Don't use this as a tool to make a diagnosis** but use it to help inform your diagnosis.

Step 6: Describe the three Ps

You are now in a powerful position to start to fully explain the separate elements of the three Ps. This is especially important in those patients with pathology who have assumed that conditions like depression or anxiety are a function of personality, or those who feel that such conditions are only possible as a result of certain life events.

On your diagram, show the patient the three Ps.

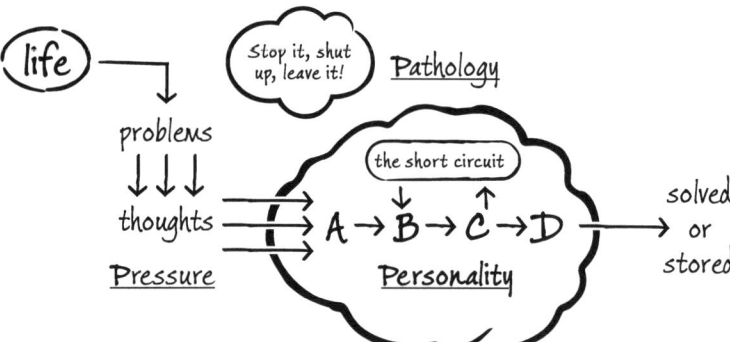

I would avoid drawing on the three Ps, as your diagram will be getting very busy. But it is very important at this stage to get several key messages across.

First, define the patient's personality as how they would normally think, behave and feel. Impress upon them the importance that this is the 'real' them. This is what the patient wants to get back, and this is what you will help them get back. Many people will offer positive features of their personality. 'I'm usually the strong one,' or 'I am the sort of person that will rationalise and I'm very analytical'.

Whereas this may have been stated by the patient as a reason they could not be 'depressed' or have 'anxiety', it is now important to show that these conditions have nothing to do with it. At this stage it's important to acknowledge, nurture and promote the patient's personality.

For example:

'Yes, I can see you are a strong-willed individual, you have shown that through various stages in your life. And this is the person we will aim to get back.'

'You say that you are the one that people in your family have come to rely on in a crisis, and you have performed that job admirably. That's the real you, that hasn't changed. Let's work to get the old you back.'

Next, talk about pressure. Explain to the patient that this represents the totality of the issues in their life which are deemed stressors. This will be the 'tap' that drip-feeds thoughts in the mind. It represents the 'traffic' through that patient's brain. At this stage, it would usually be good to give the patient examples from their own life which you will have picked up by now.

'Your debt situation is causing these thoughts to pop up into your mind – such as how you are going to find the money or what might happen if you have to sell your home.'

'You recently lost your father, and your thoughts of him are coming into your mind.'

'You have a great number of stressful events going on – the volume of thoughts going through your mind must be very high.'

You can then point out the short circuit and indicate that this is pathology. By doing this it elegantly and visually separates the illness from their personality and their life pressures. You can now show them that, as their doctor, you may not be able to change the external stressors of their life, but you can still help them by addressing the mental health disorder. Their life stressors and pressure and the thoughts associated with these will still be there; however, they won't get trapped in the short circuit.

> ### Key concepts
>
> - **The thoughts aren't the issue; the circuit is** – show the patient that the three Ps are separate things.
> - **Fixing the circuit will help them** – and this will return their normal personality, and they will be helped irrespective of whether or not their life problems can be fixed.

Step 7: Depression or anxiety, or both?

You may not be able to change the external stressors of a patient's life, but you can still help them by addressing the mental health disorder.

The following two steps will depend on your patient's specific need. You will now start to show them how different things can get stuck in the circuit and effectively cause different mental health problems. In front of you, you will have the diagram that we've drawn so far. Depending on the nature of the patient's presentation you may wish to concentrate on different types of pathologies such as anxiety or depression. However, I still find it helpful at this point to draw on several types to illustrate the fact that these different types of mental illness have so much in common with this analogy.

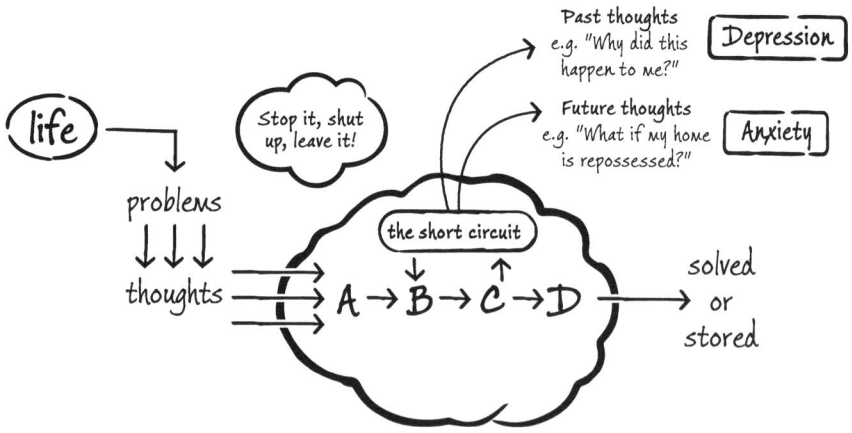

Now add to your diagram lines that come out of the short circuit. Explain that the short circuit can cause different types of thoughts to loop. Depending on the type of thought that gets stuck in the loop, different symptoms can occur. I will almost always add past events pointing to depression and future events pointing to anxiety. Depending on the circumstances you may add other lines to this, such as task-related thoughts leading to OCD. You may even add something like a thought of a past trauma leading to PTSD, or a thought about personal body image leading to an eating disorder or body dysmorphic disorder. Clearly what you do at this point will depend on the individual patient and their need. Many times I found that at this point the patient will say specifically that they often have thoughts of the future that get stuck or thoughts of the past that get stuck. This again can lend evidence to your potential diagnosis of anxiety or depression, respectively.

At this point your patient should be starting to get a clear picture of why depression and anxiety are so related to each other. As I've said previously, this can be a revelation to them when they've struggled for so long with the fact that they are being treated for depression when they feel they have anxiety, or vice versa.

Key concepts

- Add the lines to show that the thoughts stuck in the short circuit will define whether the patient gets one type of illness or another.
- Show a minimum of past for depression and future for anxiety, but add others if you need to illustrate a specific point.

Step 8: Downstream symptoms - linking physical and mental health

This step is again dependent on the specific need of you and your patient during the consultation. I will quite often add this step in when there is a specific need to explain how a mental health condition can lead to a physical health condition. More on this phenomenon is detailed in *Section 5.1.2: Another mechanism for somatic symptoms*. However, since you are drawing this diagram currently I think it's an excellent opportunity to add this correlation because it flows on very nicely. It also helps to show to the patient that in dealing with a physical health symptom such as abdominal bloating or palpitations, it may be fruitful to deal directly with the mental health issue.

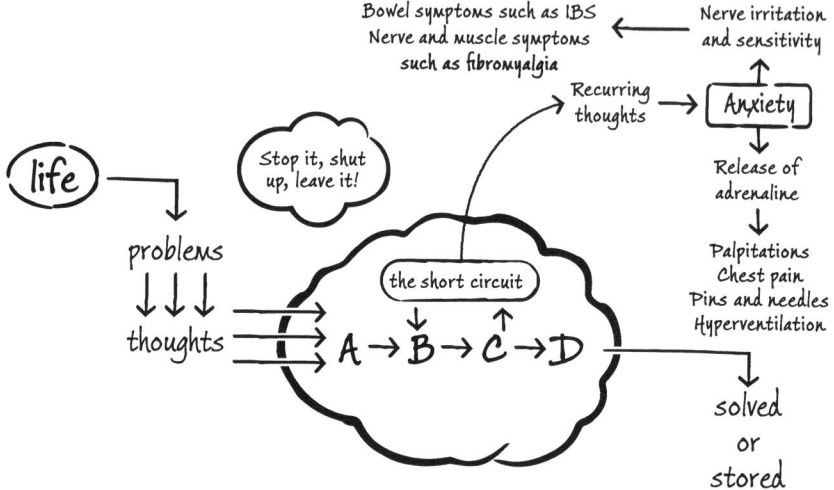

By solving the problem upstream you may be able to solve a number of downstream problems.

Following on from your arrows depicting anxiety or depression or whichever specific mental health condition you have chosen to illustrate, you can add further arrows. In this diagram I've added them to the anxiety stream.

Now you can show the patient how, at this point, other bodily functions kick in. In the diagram above I've added the release of adrenaline, nerve irritation and bowel symptoms. The adrenaline surge helps the patient understand how the short circuit loop was the first step in the eventual release of adrenaline which then gave them their cardiac-like symptoms. This is the physical manifestation of the 'flight or fight' response. Nerve irritation may be responsible, in your patient, for something like a chronic pain syndrome or fibromyalgia. Bowel symptoms could include bloating or pain and present as irritable bowel syndrome. The key message here is that the short circuit, i.e. the mental health pathology, was the first step in a chain of events that gave the patient fairly disparate and apparently unconnected physical symptoms. I've often found this simple explanation resonates extremely well with people who have struggled with this connection all their lives.

It also is worth pointing out at this point that by solving the problem upstream you may be able to solve a number of downstream problems. An example of this may be the treatment for fibromyalgia. Many fibromyalgia patients are on multiple pain-killing drugs. Often it can be the case that without these they are in too much pain to do their daily activities. However, by treating the short circuit mental health pathology in the first instance it may even reduce the need for medicines that only act further downstream. Many clinicians will recognise that once mental health is adequately treated, patients will find it much easier to reduce long-term opioid-based painkillers.

> **Key concepts**
>
> - Show that there are **specific physical manifestations of the short circuit pathology**.
> - Show the patient **how connected the mental health pathology is to the physical health pathology**.
> - Show the patient that by halting the looping, you may be able to improve a number of 'downstream' symptoms.

3.4 Summary

You have now completed your short circuit tool in the consultation. It does require a little bit of practice to get this down to a few minutes.

Practise this with your colleagues. If you are a medical student or a registrar, present this to your peer group. By doing it a number of times you will be able to do it slickly but also add your own personal twist. I created many of these diagrams over a number of years and the way I do it now, as presented above, is a combination of many attempts, some of which were less successful. When I first started doing them in the consultation, it took too long despite it being extremely helpful to myself and the patient in future visits. It was therefore impractical to do with many of the patients who I felt could benefit from it. I tried other techniques and found that I had not necessarily fully or adequately conveyed my meaning to the patient. After many iterations, I eventually found that this style produced consistent results in a short consultation time and with a high degree of precision and reproducibility.

Nevertheless we all work differently. Each consultation will have a different need and tone associated with it. You will need to adjust your explanation for each patient. Depending on why you started doing the short circuit tool in the first place, you may want to spend a little more or less time on specific steps.

For example, with the patient who believes that they cannot have a mental illness due to the strength of their personality, or the patient that may feel upset that their sense of self has been marred by a mental health diagnosis, you should concentrate on separating the personality from the pathology in your diagram. For patients who feel that they can never feel better until their life circumstances change, you should concentrate on showing them that whilst their life circumstances may be the same after medical treatment, you have still treated their pathology. This will be of great comfort to them and give them hope.

3.5 Worked examples

3.5.1 A depressed patient who doesn't believe in depression

> **Case study - Mr Holmes**
>
> Mr Holmes is an ex-serviceman who has worked as a self-employed management consultant since leaving the Forces. He presents with typical symptoms of depression, including sleep loss, loss of libido, irritability and a persistent low mood. However, he does not feel that such a diagnosis could apply to him due to his strength of character, his renowned ability to cope with stressful situations and his distinguished army career.

Here Mr Holmes' doctor recognises the signs and symptoms of a possible depression diagnosis; however, they also recognise that Mr Holmes has a misconception of depression, in that he feels that it only applies to certain 'types' of people and in fact is not a medical illness but a personality trait.

The doctor explains that they will show Mr Holmes a different way to look at the illness of depression which may help him understand it better. The doctor starts with a short circuit diagram, concentrating on:

- reinforcing Mr Holmes' sense of self – his resilience and strength of character
- showing that the depression (as visualised by the short circuit) is a separate thing to personality
- showing that depression exists as a real pathology (see *Section 4.2*)
- exploring the nature of the thoughts that get trapped in the short circuit – past or future
- explaining that if the diagnosis is indeed depression, by breaking the short circuit, Mr Holmes' symptoms can dramatically improve and he can start to regain his old self.

After making a formal diagnosis using approved means, the doctor then goes on to explain the treatments available for depression (see *Section 4.2: Focus on depression* and *Chapter 6: Treating the patient*) before developing a plan together with Mr Holmes.

3.5.2 An anxious patient with high levels of life stressors

Case study – Mrs Pearson

Mrs Pearson is a teacher who looks after learning disabled children. Her school is going through a large-scale restructure and possible merger. She feels bullied by her boss. At the same time, she has been suffering with IBS and has had numerous GI investigations, although she has a strong suspicion that this is something more serious. She presents with symptoms of anxiety, including restlessness, recurring thoughts of negative events and sleep disturbance. She feels that the doctor can help her by re-referring her for repeat GI investigations and writing to her school about the possible bullying.

Here Mrs Pearson's doctor recognises the signs and symptoms of a possible anxiety diagnosis. However, they also recognise that Mrs Pearson feels that her symptoms are wholly due to her life circumstances – she feels that if her boss were to change, she would not have her current symptoms, and if she could be reassured by further GI tests, she could feel more confident and no longer have her emotional symptoms.

The doctor explains that they will show Mrs Pearson a way to look at the illness of anxiety which may help her understand that it can occur with or without the life pressures she is under. The doctor starts with a short circuit diagram, concentrating on:

- acknowledging Mrs Pearson's set of life pressures
- showing that the short circuit is a separate thing to her pressure and stress
- explaining that whilst she has a lot of life pressure and stressors coming into her mind, there may also be a 'short circuit', therefore creating her anxiety symptoms
- exploring the nature of the thoughts that get trapped in the short circuit – past or future
- explaining that if the diagnosis is indeed anxiety, by breaking the short circuit, she may see a dramatic improvement in her mental health, even though her life stressors (i.e. her work situation) may still be there.

After making a formal diagnosis using approved means, the doctor then goes on to explain the treatments available for anxiety (see *Section 4.1: Focus on anxiety* and *Chapter 6: Treating the patient*) before developing a plan together with Mrs Pearson.

If the doctor is satisfied that the GI symptoms are indeed secondary to IBS, they may go on to explain that by treating the anxiety, Mrs Pearson may see an improvement in her physical symptoms in a way that repeating investigations would not do.

○

Chapter 4

Mental illnesses in detail

4.1 Focus on anxiety

> **What you'll learn in this section**
> This section describes the classification, epidemiology, diagnosis and treatment of anxiety as a disorder.
>
> **How this helps**
> Anxiety is a commonly seen illness and clinicians should have a good grasp of its diagnosis and management.

Anxiety is not a single entity. In ICD-11 it is listed under 'Mental, behavioural or neurodevelopmental disorders' with the heading 'anxiety or fear-related disorders'. There are a further eleven subcategories, including generalised anxiety disorder (GAD), agoraphobia, selective mutism and social anxiety.

Anxiety is one of the single most common mental health conditions.

In reality these different categorisations do not occur entirely in isolation. Patients will often present with a collection of symptoms which will fall into one or a number of these categories. It is important not to see these as completely separate. Moreover, they are a useful way of categorising a set of the patient's symptoms with a view to giving them a specific treatment plan. It is very easy for patients to become concerned with whether they have one diagnosis or another. This labelling is rarely helpful for the patient to come to terms with the illness or have a good understanding of their underlying condition.

Nevertheless it is useful to know and understand, as a clinician, that there are a number of different syndromic groups that patients with an anxiety disorder can fall into.

4.1.1 Classifications of anxiety

ICD-11 has the following subcategories of anxiety disorders:

- Generalised anxiety disorder (GAD)
- Panic disorder
- Agoraphobia
- Specific phobia
- Social anxiety disorder
- Separation anxiety disorder
- Selective mutism
- Substance-induced anxiety disorders
- Hypochondriasis
- Secondary anxiety syndrome.

The breakdown is partially based on the specific anxiety trigger (such as social anxiety or specific phobia), or on the specific type of symptomatic reaction (mutism or panic disorder), or on the aetiology (e.g. substance-induced).

Since these subsets are fluid and not entirely specific, no classification can define them perfectly satisfactorily along a single characteristic.

4.1.2 Epidemiology

Anxiety is one of the single most common mental health conditions in the population. It is also one of the most common chronic health conditions overall. The lifetime prevalence of those who experience anything within the anxiety spectrum is over 20%, and within a single year any random individual has over 15% chance of suffering from an anxiety disorder. The highest prevalence amongst these conditions is social anxiety disorder and specific phobias, followed closely by GAD and panic disorders. Anxiety disorders, particularly GAD, are more prevalent in females and have a peak incidence in the 4th to 6th decade of life. However, they are present in both sexes, all ages and across all other demographic splits. A number of factors are associated with an increased risk of developing an anxiety disorder:

- Positive family history of anxiety or other mental health conditions
- Personal history of anxiety in childhood or adolescence
- History of life events causing high levels of distress
- Female sex
- Personal experience of abuse or other trauma
- Chronic physical health condition such as cardiovascular disease or diabetes
- Substance dependence or abuse
- Chronic pain.

4.1.3 Screening tools and presentation

The first step in making a diagnosis of anxiety or indeed any other mental health problem is being alert in recognising it. There will be occasions where patients come in and give a very clear indication that they feel as though anxiety is at play. However, many other times anxiety as a pathology will present itself as a set of physical or emotional symptoms.

Consider an anxiety disorder when the patient is showing specific emotional or physical symptoms of anxiety (see section below). Be particularly alert when the patient has been in a number of times seeking reassurances, even after these reassurances have been given.

As described in previous chapters there are a number of barriers to opening the dialogue about anxiety. Consider the three Ps model. Many people will incorrectly assume that anxiety is a function of personality or simply a function of their life pressures. The notion of anxiety, along with many other mental health conditions, is shrouded in stigma. Many people would much prefer a physical diagnosis to a mental health diagnosis and as such, anxiety may remain undiagnosed for many years.

If your suspicion of anxiety is raised through the signs and symptoms that your patient is presenting with it is necessary to skilfully and delicately raise the issue of anxiety. Given that this is a very stigmatised condition it's important that you do this carefully. Be empathetic and consider one of the following openings:

- *'Are these feelings of worry making it difficult to live your life? Is it worth exploring this?'*
- *'Is the worry about your health stopping you from sleeping? Do you wish you could worry less?'*
- *'Are you avoiding doing things to stop yourself getting anxious?'*
- *'Anxiety can be a very distressing and unpleasant condition. Do you want to talk about how we can address the anxiety?'*
- *'I wonder if you might be suffering from something called anxiety. Would you like me to help you with this?'*

Remember that even if anxiety is there as an underlying pathology, the patient may not wish to explore this. Remember the relationship between personality, pressure and pathology. Remember that due to underlying stigma patients may confuse the pathology of anxiety with the notion of their own personality or the current pressure (or lack of pressure) that their life is under. As described in previous chapters, this is a good time to start the short circuit tool if appropriate.

There are alternative methods of picking up anxiety other than the diagnostic suspicion of a presentation. There are some screening tools available. The shortest and quickest of these is the generalised anxiety disorder scale (GAD-2). Its use during a primary care consultation is not well supported through study. However, the screening tool could be used in other patient contact situations such as a nurse-led follow-up clinic for a chronic physical disease such as diabetes. The GAD-2 test asks two simple questions, each scoring from 0 to 3.

GAD-2

'Over the last 2 weeks, how often have you been bothered by the following problems?'

- Q1 – Feeling nervous, anxious or on edge (score 0–3)
- Q2 – Being unable to stop or control worrying (score 0-3)

Scores:

- 0 – Not at all
- 1 – Several days
- 2 – More than half the days
- 3 – Nearly every day

A score of 3 or more would indicate a further exploration of anxiety.

The GAD-7 tool is also available – and can be found widely online (e.g. at patient.info[1]) – and this is usually done by the patient in their own time. Some clinicians use sequential scores on a GAD-7 to assess progress of their patient. It can be repeated after a minimum of 2 weeks. This does have a stronger evidence base – especially for GAD. [2]

4.1.4 Emotional and behavioural symptoms

The emotional and behavioural characteristics of anxiety are given in the table below, split by subcategory. However, all types of anxiety share the same core features:

- an uncontrollable excess of anxiety and worry
- recurring looping thoughts about future situations
- a propensity towards feeling fear and the avoidance of possible negative outcomes.

The symptom set associated with each of the subcategories is what defines them, so these are given separately in the table:

---

[1] https://patient.info/doctor/generalised-anxiety-disorder-assessment-gad-7

[2] Swinson, R.P. (2006) The GAD-7 scale was accurate for diagnosing generalised anxiety disorder. *Evid Based Med.*, **11(6):** 184.

Subcategory	Triggers/affected thoughts and scenarios	Symptoms
Generalised anxiety disorder (GAD)	Not specific and can occur in many different scenarios	Often persistent, low-level recurring thoughts throughout the day with some worse periods Looping thoughts, 'what ifs' with many different future scenarios playing out Often associated with a number of physical symptoms such as headaches, pain and insomnia (see below)
Panic disorder	Sometimes recognisable triggers exist; however, panic episodes can come on without triggers	Whilst GAD is associated with low-level persistent symptoms, panic disorder is usually associated with short-lived intense symptoms lasting up to one hour at a time (panic attacks) Physical symptoms are usually intense and often adrenaline-mediated; these can include palpitations, breathlessness and chest pain The patient will often interpret these signs as catastrophic and have intense fear for their own life Once a single panic attack has occurred, the patient will have recurring thoughts and fears of further episodes (secondary anxiety)
Agoraphobia	Being in crowds, open spaces, outside the home or when using public transport	Recurrent or looping thoughts occur when the patient is in these trigger situations Fear of inability to escape occurs, with adrenaline-mediated physical symptoms Avoidance behaviours result in significant limitations to life Panic attacks occur when the patient is in triggered situations In extreme situations patients are unable to leave the home, sometimes for many years

Subcategory	Triggers/affected thoughts and scenarios	Symptoms
Specific phobia	Very precise triggers such as spiders, flying, needles or dental surgery	Patients may not show any physical or emotional signs of anxiety in the absence of the specific trigger When the trigger is present they can often develop panic disorder-like symptoms; the perception of threat is vastly disproportional to the real level of danger Patients will develop avoidance strategies which can sometimes affect their ability to live life and conduct daily activities
Social anxiety disorder	Meeting new people Being amongst unfamiliar groups Eating in public	Recurrent thoughts of being negatively judged by other people Fear of being observed by others Often panic attack-like symptoms can occur when the trigger criteria are met Avoidance behaviours such as being unable to meet new people Negative impact on education and work performance which further exacerbates the underlying condition in a vicious circle
Separation anxiety disorder	Separation from a caregiver or receiver	Most often found in babies and children; however, can extend into adolescence Can occur in adults, such as mothers separated from their babies or young adults going to university Symptoms can present similar to GAD but with acute panic disorder-like episodes on top Thoughts can be recurrent of bad events happening to themselves or the person they are separated from Avoidance behaviours are common

Subcategory	Triggers/affected thoughts and scenarios	Symptoms
Selective mutism	Can be associated with specific triggers such as public speaking or be more generalised with no specific trigger	This is a less common manifestation of anxiety and is usually diagnosed in childhood Adults can also have this following on from childhood illness, or develop it during adulthood Can occur in conjunction with a post-traumatic stress disorder but most cases are not associated with specific trauma or abuse The ability to vocalise sounds is completely diminished during attacks Often misdiagnosed as shyness in children Usually needs speech and language therapy as well as treatment for the anxiety
Substance-induced anxiety	Triggered by ingestion of recreational drug	Symptoms can include those of panic disorder predominantly Substances implicated can include cannabis, alcohol, amphetamines or cocaine Some drugs can include dissociative and hallucinogenic symptoms, such as ketamine or phencyclidine (PCP).
Hypochondriasis/health anxiety	Physical health symptoms of any description	There is a preoccupation and intense cycling thoughts about having or developing a serious medical illness These thoughts will persist despite reassurance or testing which shows evidence to the contrary Can cause frequent checking of symptoms and signs including home monitoring of e.g. blood pressure Conducting tests may relieve anxiety temporarily; however, often new recurrent thoughts appear

Subcategory	Triggers/affected thoughts and scenarios	Symptoms
Secondary anxiety disorder	Triggered by another underlying chronic health condition, including anxiety itself	The recurrent thoughts are about the primary health condition; e.g. a patient with epilepsy can develop anxiety as a result of the fear of the consequences of the epilepsy There could also be recurrent fear of the effects of the anxiety itself – patients can become afraid that they're worrying too much; the anxiety thereby breeds further anxiety in a positive feedback loop

Referring back to the short circuit diagram, where different patients get different thoughts 'trapped' in the short circuit, you can think of the 'triggers' in the above table as the types of thoughts that get trapped in the circuit. The different subsections of anxiety are associated with different types of thoughts that have a propensity to get trapped.

4.1.5 Physical symptoms

Anxiety can have clear and distinct physical symptoms associated with it. These are broken into two categories. The first is directly mediated by the release of adrenaline and cortisol. The second category includes a number of syndromes which do not as yet have any definitive proven biochemical associations but are clearly linked to anxiety.

Adrenaline-mediated symptoms

Adrenaline is a key life-sustaining hormone. One of its purposes is to prepare the body for dangerous situations. In evolutionary terms the human body is designed to respond to serious life-threatening stress in a preordained physical way. For the vast majority of human evolution this has been the appropriate response to most danger. The history of modern humanity as farmers or people living in towns and cities with contemporary lifestyles is far too short on an evolutionary timescale to have made any real impact on our underlying biology. We are still designed, like all mammals, to react with a specific set of physical changes when our brains sense that our lives are in danger.

Adrenaline and cortisol, along with other hormones, are released once the danger alarms are triggered. Adrenaline is produced predominantly by the adrenal gland but is also made in the medulla oblongata in the brain. It causes:

- stimulation of beta-adrenergic receptors in the heart to increase contractility and heart rate
- relaxation of smooth muscles in the lungs to enhance inspiratory capacity
- stimulation of the liver to break down glycogen into glucose to provide quick energy
- contraction of the arteries in the skin to divert blood flow
- contraction of muscles in the skin causing hairs to raise
- diversion of blood away from bowel and other non-essential organs
- increase in certain neurotransmitter pathways in the brain.

Symptomatic effects of adrenaline:

- Sharpening of the mind and senses
- Dilation of the pupils, allowing more light in
- Increased pulse rate and a possible sense of palpitations
- Tension in the muscles in readiness to run or fight
- Increased sweat production
- Breathing more deeply and rapidly to increase oxygen transfer
- Tingling in the peripheral nerves such as fingers – 'pins and needles'
- Dryness of the mucous membranes as secretions reduce
- Bowel symptoms, such as the urgency to defecate or abdominal cramping.

In anxiety disorders one of the key fundamental features is that the body mistakenly perceives a much greater degree of danger than the actual threat. For example, in an individual with phobic disorder the real danger associated with the flying is far less than that perceived by the mind of the patient. Equally in a patient with a social anxiety disorder or agoraphobia the real threat to themselves in a social gathering outside of the home is far less than that perceived.

Since the perception of danger is there, adrenaline and cortisol are released. The patient's body will enter a 'flight or fight' mode and the constellation of symptoms associated with adrenaline release listed above will ensue. This is analogous to a car alarm going off persistently and inappropriately when there is no car theft taking place.

One of the key fundamental features is that the body mistakenly perceives a much greater degree of danger than the actual threat.

Differential diagnosis of these symptoms

The physical symptoms of anxiety are similar to the following and care should be taken to eliminate these from your differential.

Cardiovascular

- Angina and myocardial infarction (dyspnoea, chest pain, palpitations)
- Cardiac arrhythmias (palpitations, dyspnoea, syncope)
- Cardiac valvular disease, e.g. mitral valve prolapse (dyspnoea)

Respiratory

- Pulmonary embolus (dyspnoea, tachypnoea, chest pain)
- Asthma and other obtrusive respiratory disorders (breathlessness, wheezing)

Endocrine

- Hyperthyroidism (e.g. palpitations, tachycardia, heat intolerance)
- Hypoglycaemia (sweats, palpitations, dizziness)
- Phaeochromocytoma (e.g. headache, palpitations, breathlessness, hypertension)
- Hypoparathyroidism (e.g. muscle cramps, paraesthesia)

Neurological

- Transient ischaemic attacks (TIAs)
- Seizures.

The above list is not exhaustive and it is outside the scope of this book to detail all possible differential diagnoses of symptoms. However, care should be taken not to overlook a possible cardiac, respiratory, endocrine or neurological cause of the patient's symptoms.

Other physical symptoms

In *Section 5.1.2: Another mechanism for somatic symptoms*, a description is given of how anxiety could theoretically cause any number of physical symptoms. This can be described as somatisation. However, several syndromic sets of symptoms commonly appear in anxiety disorders. These are given specific individual consideration in their own sections in *Chapter 5: Physical illness with mental health connections*. However, the following physical symptoms can be quite consistent across different types and forms of anxiety:

- Memory difficulties (brain fog)
- Sleep disturbance (difficulty getting to sleep or regular waking during the night)
- Difficulty in concentrating or making decisions.

These are specific syndromic associations of anxiety:

Irritable bowel syndrome

- Abdominal bloating and pain
- Changes to bowel habit: diarrhoea or constipation or swinging from one to the other
- The sensation of being full quickly
- Urgency of defecation, e.g. needing to go several times in the morning
- Abdominal pain that relieves after defecation.

See *Section 5.3: Irritable bowel syndrome*.

Fibromyalgia

- Increased sensitivity to pain – particularly in the joints, muscle and skin

- Extreme tiredness and fatigue
- Muscle stiffness
- Difficulty sleeping
- Headaches
- A sensation of swelling of the joints without there being real swelling.

See *Section 5.2: Fibromyalgia.*

Chronic fatigue syndrome

- Sleep problems
- Intense overwhelming fatigue and tiredness
- Headaches and a sore throat or sore glands that are not swollen
- Difficulty with concentration, memory and thinking
- Flu-like symptoms
- Dizziness or feeling sick.

See *Section 5.5: Chronic fatigue syndrome.*

The physical symptoms of the pathology of anxiety can be vast and often difficult to attribute to anxiety as a layperson. It is extremely easy to see that symptoms as disparate as memory loss, joint pain and diarrhoea would not obviously lead an average intelligent layperson to believe that they are suffering from an anxiety disorder.

It is therefore fairly easy to see how resistance to the diagnosis of anxiety in a patient with these symptoms could occur. It is therefore vital for the clinician to have within their skill set the ability to show patients how these physical and mental things can be connected. The short circuit tool can be extremely useful in this scenario.

4.1.6 The short circuit analogy for anxiety

Remember that the short circuit tool is a mechanism to help the patient 'see' the mental health disorder. Its purpose is predominantly to help reduce stigma, help the patient connect physical symptoms to a mental health disorder, and help them separate their own sense of self from the diagnosis of a mental illness.

Future problem thought

- What if this mole is cancer?
- What if I can't pay my bills?
- What if the plane comes down mid flight?
- What if those people laugh at me?

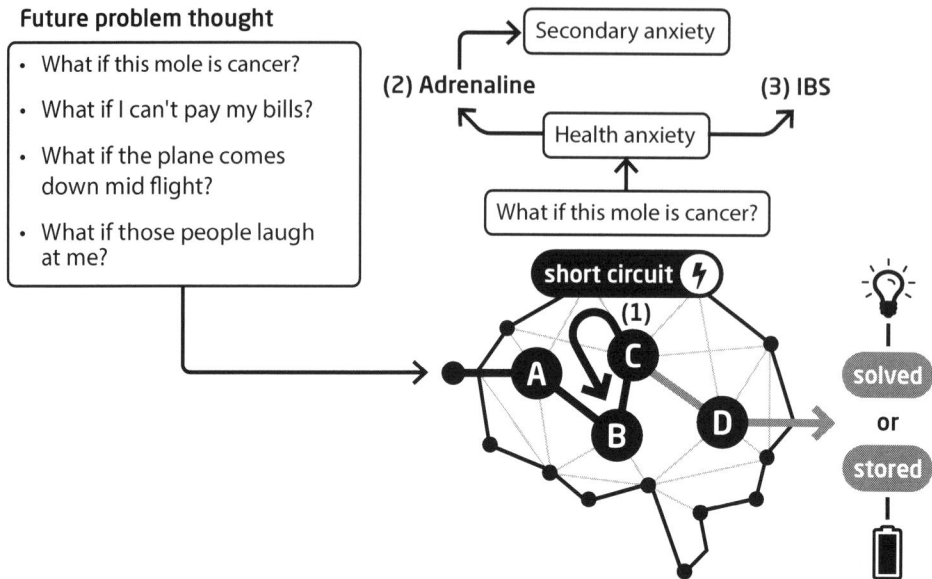

In the short circuit description, as shown in the diagram above, any normal person has a number of thoughts entering their mind at any one time. It is perfectly normal, for example, to wonder if a mole could be cancerous. Many people have thought about whether a plane may come down in flight. It is quite common to be concerned about what people may think of you. The thoughts themselves do not represent the anxiety in the short circuit model – it is an error in the circuitry causing certain normal thoughts to loop. Remember that it is only certain thoughts that loop; others flow through normally, as indicated by the arrows beyond C and the fact that these are still solved or stored.

When an anxiety disorder exists, however, the short circuit is there and pushes selected thoughts into a loop. Certain thoughts can now short circuit back from C to B and become trapped. A common feature of all types of anxiety disorder is that the thoughts that are trapped are about possible future events. Depending on the type of thought which is stuck, different types of anxiety disorder can be categorised.

Type	Thoughts that get trapped in the short circuit
Generalised anxiety disorder	Trapping of many different types of thoughts of future events
Health anxiety/ hypochondriasis	Only thoughts related specifically to a health concern (as in diagram above)
Phobias	Only thoughts relating to a specific physical thing or scenario; other thoughts generally do not get stuck

When trying to help the patient visualise the illness, you can point to the short circuit on the diagram. The existence of the short circuit means they have the mental health symptoms. The type of thought that gets trapped in the short circuit gets them the particular syndrome. Once the short circuit exists, there are a number of 'downstream' effects. In the diagram above this includes the adrenaline surge, IBS and secondary anxiety.

Using the short circuit diagram you can also identify a number of treatment targets. These are shown on the diagram, in this case, as numbers 1, 2 and 3.

Treatment of the patient with the mental health disorder is considered in detail in *Chapter 6: Treating the patient*. However, from this simple diagram you can identify and point out these three targets. Treatment to target 1 will involve breaking the short circuit. Treatments which affect this target will include simple lifestyle measures, therapies such as cognitive behavioural therapy (CBT) or medications such as selective serotonin reuptake inhibitors (SSRIs). You can demonstrate on this diagram how treating at this target will potentially have a benefit on all further downstream symptoms.

The patient can also be treated at target 2 in this instance. Treatments here will aim to reduce the overall effect of the adrenaline surge, such as the use of a beta-blocker. These treatments may not stop the short circuit cognitive symptoms but will stop anything downstream of that target point. This has a clear benefit of reducing the symptoms of a panic attack. Treatment at this target could include an improvement in the secondary anxiety symptoms. Secondary anxiety in this patient may come as a result of the physical symptoms with the adrenaline surge, i.e. the mind races, then the heart races, then the mind races, etc.

A third target, 3, is indicated on the diagram. In this case the patient is suffering from IBS. There are a number of medicines specifically for IBS which can improve symptoms. These are detailed in *Section 5.3: Irritable bowel syndrome*. Again, these therapies will be good in stopping the downstream physical symptoms of anxiety but will not play a part in improving the cognitive symptoms caused by the short circuit in the first place. It may be extremely helpful to show the patient these treatment targets to help them understand your rationale for choosing or recommending a treatment. It may also be extremely helpful in helping them understand why a drug such as an antidepressant can be so helpful in tackling physical symptoms.

4.1.7 Causes of anxiety

Occasionally, you will be asked :

'But what is the cause of my anxiety?'

This is a perfectly reasonable and intelligent question. However, the answer is complex and in many respects not entirely satisfactorily complete.

If you have taken the patient through the short circuit model you may be asked:

'I understand that thoughts are becoming trapped in the short circuit but why is the short circuit there in the first place?'

This line of questioning is natural for any type of physical or mental health long-term condition. Patients will quite rightly ask why they have asthma or why they have diabetes.

Many patients, quite understandably, spend a great deal of time looking for a cause for their mental illness.

At the time of writing there is still no single cause identified. There are a number of associations which give us clues as to the possible aetiology. The biopsychosocial model is still the most acceptable explanation. But even with this there will be many cases where the aetiology is unknown or random. Some patients will have a genetic component, whilst others will have some obvious traumatic trigger. However, a very large component will have no obvious cause. In the interested and motivated patient you should discuss the causes as listed below. However, for a short discussion on the subject, a suggested narrative is given in *Section 2.1.4*.

Many patients, quite understandably, spend a great deal of time looking for a cause. This is a perfectly natural human instinct. In some cases a specific cause or likely cause can be found, and this can give the patient some degree of comfort and answer. However, when there is no obvious single cause this journey can lead to frustration. For some patients it can make them vulnerable to particular people, websites or social media groups which purport to give them a definitive cause.

Biopsychosocial model

Sometimes one or more of the following biological, social or psychological factors are implicated. Sometimes there is a combination of a number of factors, whilst at other times none of these are present.

Biological:

- Female sex
- Family history of anxiety or other psychiatric disorders
- Substance dependence
- Chronic pain or chronic physical health conditions

Psychological:

- Physical or emotional trauma
- Childhood abuse or maltreatment
- Bullying and victimisation
- Excessive parental pressure during childhood

Social:

- Lack of personal social networks, such as being divorced or separated
- Life events, such as moving home or bereavement
- Unemployment

- Domestic violence
- Parental and home problems such as alcoholism, poor mental health or domestic violence.

The absence of any of the above factors does not exclude anxiety as a diagnosis. Equally the presence of many or all of the above factors does not always mean that the individual suffers with anxiety disorder.

Pinning the 'cause' or 'blame' of an anxiety disorder on a single cause may provide a false impression to the patient. They may falsely attribute their condition to people from their past or take some false hope that by removing certain things in their lives they will be cured.

4.1.8 Management

Before you start any 'management' of anxiety, you should convince yourself that the patient has understood the diagnosis and has a good concept of 'what' you are trying to treat. If you have used the short circuit tool, you can tell them that you are trying to break the short circuit, therefore enabling all the thoughts that arise through their life problems to flow through their minds without bouncing persistently between B and C. They will still have their problems in life and they will still have worrying thoughts, but the thoughts will not be all-consuming. If the treatment is successful, they are likely to see their real personality shine through again.

Patients undergoing any form of medical treatment are more likely to be compliant and more likely to see success if they are fully invested in the plan, feel part of it and have been centrally involved in its inception. Starting treatment for a mental health disorder in a patient who either doesn't believe they have it or doesn't understand it is much more likely to fail. This is where, I believe, the short circuit tool can add significantly to the patient experience.

All patients should be encouraged to adopt self-management techniques.

As with the management of any mental health disorder, treatment should be offered to the patient in a stepwise fashion and in full collaboration with the patient. However, the steps should not be rigidly applied to every patient. It is generally better to have a good mastery of each of these treatment modalities so that you can apply them more personally to the patient in front of you.

When offering treatments it's important to fully educate the patient about the pros and cons of each treatment. Be aware that a number of stigmas or preconceptions may exist about any type of mental health treatment, including talking therapies and medicines. Often patients may choose the wrong type of therapy based on an incorrect assumption.

NICE suggests a four-step approach. The table below is adapted from the guidelines, originally published in 2011 but updated in 2019, on generalised anxiety disorder; however, it can be reasonably used as a basis for many different types of anxiety presentation.

	Who is this for?	Nature of the intervention
Step 1	All known and suspected presentations of GAD	Identification and assessment; education about anxiety and treatment options; active monitoring
Step 2	Diagnosed anxiety that has not improved after education and active monitoring in primary care	Low-intensity psychological interventions: individual non-facilitated self-help, individual guided self-help and psychoeducational groups
Step 3	Anxiety with an inadequate response to step 2 interventions or marked functional impairment	Choice of a high-intensity psychological intervention (CBT/applied relaxation) or a drug treatment
Step 4	Complex treatment-refractory anxiety and very marked functional impairment, such as self-neglect or a high risk of self-harm	Highly specialist treatment, such as complex drug and/or psychological treatment regimens; input from multi-agency teams, crisis services, day hospitals or inpatient care

Step 1

Education and self-management
All patients should be encouraged to adopt self-management techniques. These help the patient feel empowered and are useful throughout the spectrum of anxiety disorders.

Self-management techniques can include:

- lifestyle measures such as exercise and healthy eating
- self-help approaches through books or websites
- mindfulness and meditation techniques.

Step 2

See *Section 6.4* for a detailed consideration of CBT.

Low-intensity psychological therapies

Low-intensity therapies are fundamentally a way of getting a better cost–benefit outcome for more patients. Since these methods require fewer therapists per patient, they can be deployed over a much larger patient cohort – particularly those who may not need the intensity of dedicated one-to-one sessions. Psychological therapies considered as low-intensity are:

- Guided self-administered CBT
  - this should be supported by a trained facilitator but the patient does much of the reading and personal reflection
  - usually consists of 5–7 weekly or fortnightly face-to-face or telephone sessions, each lasting 20–30 minutes
- Psychoeducational groups
  - these are group sessions based on CBT
  - they should be conducted by trained practitioners
  - they will usually have a ratio of one therapist to about twelve participants
  - these are not suitable for certain forms of anxiety, such as social anxiety disorder
- Computerised CBT
  - this can be used instead of face-to-face guided CBT
  - may be more accessible and convenient for some
  - evidence is currently lacking for its effectiveness.

Step 3

After step 2, NICE advises high-intensity psychological intervention and/or pharmacological treatments.

High-intensity psychological therapy

High-intensity therapy differs from low-intensity in that it is usually done in a one-to-one setting with a trained therapist. It is based on the principles of CBT. The therapist will have regular supervision to monitor fidelity to the treatment mode and use routine outcome measures and ensure that the patient is involved in reviewing the efficacy of the treatment.

Unlike the low-intensity version, here the patient will normally have 12–15 weekly sessions (fewer if the person recovers sooner; more if clinically required), each lasting one hour.

Pharmacological therapies

See *Section 6.5* for a detailed consideration of pharmacological therapies that may have:

- long-term anxiety treatment effects:
  - SSRIs
  - SNRIs
  - tricyclic antidepressants
  - anticonvulsants
- short-term benefit only:
  - benzodiazepines
  - beta-blockers.

A number of treatment options are available. Before embarking on any drug therapy, it is important that you educate and inform the patient. Each therapy is given thorough individual consideration in *Chapter 6: Treating the patient*, including the important patient counselling and discussion.

Long-term treatments

The single most ubiquitous drug used to treat anxiety is the SSRI, followed by selective serotonin-noradrenaline reuptake inhibitors (SNRIs) and tricyclic antidepressants (TCAs). The SSRI should be the first-line treatment for almost all patients. Exceptions may include those who have previously failed to show improvement on these in the past or those who have had significant adverse effects.

Anticonvulsants such as pregabalin can be considered second-line agents for patients who have not responded adequately.

Benzodiazepines

Benzodiazepines do not have a role in the treatment of anxiety disorders other than in the very short term. However, they do remain an important part of the armoury in the treatment of acute severe anxiety episodes. Patients in crisis may benefit from these.

When offering drugs such as diazepam, you should satisfy yourself that they will only be needed in the short term. Only prescribe small quantities. If the underlying condition is not likely to improve in the short term then benzodiazepines may not be recommended.

Beta-blockers

Beta-blockers do not have any cognitive effects and therefore should not be considered a treatment for anxiety per se. They can reduce the physical symptoms associated with the adrenergic overdrive in certain forms of anxiety, such as panic disorder.

Treating physical symptoms

Treatments for anxiety can also include those that act on downstream effects such as IBS. These can include medicine such as antispasmodics. Whilst these medicines will not have a direct impact on the cognitive effects of anxiety, they may help with the secondary anxiety symptoms and feedback loops.

Treatments for anxiety can also include those that act on downstream effects such as IBS.

See *Sections 5.2: Fibromyalgia*; *5.3: IBS*; *5.4: Chronic pain syndrome* and *5.5: Chronic fatigue syndrome* for more information.

Step 4

At step 4, you should be involving secondary care services through a referral.

Many primary care physicians will have their own threshold for referral, but consider the following as reasonable criteria on which to request a specialist opinion:

- Patients at very high risk of self-neglect or self-harm as a result of their anxiety
- Patients who maintain a very high level of functional distress despite at least two different forms of therapy offered (e.g. SSRI followed by SNRI or anticonvulsant)

- Patients who have failed to respond to dual therapy (e.g. CBT + SSRI)
- Patients who may require pharmacological adjunctive therapy.

4.1.9 Course and prognosis

The prognosis and expected course can vary with the type of anxiety the patient suffers. The most common types, social anxiety and generalised anxiety disorder, should generally be considered chronic conditions which fluctuate in severity. Other factors which influence prognosis include comorbidity with other psychiatric and physical health illness, and substance abuse.

It should also be noted that many patients present to the medical profession after suffering for many years without any intervention.

Conclusive numbers to predict the outcomes are difficult to come by due to the heterogeneity of the illness and the multifactorial nature of the likelihood of treatment success. Nevertheless, the following may be a useful guide to share with your patients.

No intervention/ treatment	Patients with a diagnosed anxiety who have no intervention, even at step 1, are generally unlikely to improve. Many patients will have lived in this state for a number of years before intervention of some description.
Step 2–3 CBT	High-intensity CBT can produce remission in 30–50% of patients
SSRIs	Studies vary – remission rates from 38 to 60%

Many anxiety disorders can be considered chronic illnesses, often lifelong, with a remitting and relapsing course. Hence patients with a prior history of mental illness may be offered longer courses of medication such as SSRIs, and for some these can continue to be prescribed as long-term prophylactic drugs.

4.2 Focus on depression

What you'll learn in this section
This section describes the classification, epidemiology, diagnosis and treatment of depression as a disorder.

How this helps
Depression is a commonly seen illness and clinicians should have a good grasp of its diagnosis and management.

4.2.1 Classifications of depression

Using the ICD-11 classifications, depression, in contrast to anxiety, has fewer categories. The categorisations of depression are predominantly around the chronicity of the presentation rather than subdivisions based on symptomatic type of the depression. Depression, unlike anxiety, seems to have a more generally uniform set of symptoms across different patients. However, the presence of psychosis in severe depression puts it in a separate ICD-11 category.

These are:

- Single depressive episode (with or without psychosis)
- Recurrent depressive episode (with or without psychosis)
- Dysthymic disorder
- Mixed depressive and anxiety disorder.

4.2.2 Epidemiology

The UN World Health Organization (WHO) recognises depression as the leading cause of disability worldwide. Between 4 and 5% of the global population suffers with depression[3]. This number has

---

[3] Global Burden of Disease Study 2013 Collaborators (2015) Global, regional, and national incidence, prevalence, and years lived with disability for 301 acute and chronic diseases and injuries in 188 countries, 1990–2013: a systematic analysis for the Global Burden of Disease Study 2013. *Lancet*, **386(9995):** 743–800.

shown a strong and steady increase over the last 10–15 years. It is unclear, however, whether this is a true effect or the result of better detection. In the UK, NHS Digital regularly publishes population data for mental health. According to these figures, nearly 20% of the population has suffered with signs and symptoms of depression[4]. Similar to the global picture, this has steadily increased over the last 5 years. This percentage is higher among females than males.

The adult psychiatric morbidity survey[5], conducted by the Office for National Statistics and NHS Digital, found that depression was most strongly associated with certain demographics. These include black women, adults under the age of 60 who lived alone, women who lived in large households, adults not in employment, those in receipt of benefits and those who smoked cigarettes. These associations are in keeping with increased social disadvantage and poverty being associated with higher risk of mental health disorders.

4.2.3 Screening tools and presentation

Depression can present itself in a multitude of ways and in a multitude of settings; hence the development of a screening tool which can help any healthcare practitioner to conduct a quick simple screen.

NICE guidelines[6] for recognition and management of depression, originally published in 2009 with regular updates, stop short of recommending screening as a national programme but they do highlight the importance of being vigilant to the possibility of depression. It is important to be alert for patients, particularly when they have a history of depression or any chronic physical health problem which is known to be associated.

The PHQ-2 tool is a screening tool based on the first two questions of the PHQ-9 (see *Section 4.2.7*). This has been abbreviated further to give a yes/no two-question screening tool and has been

[4] https://digital.nhs.uk
[5] NHS Digital (2014) *Adult Psychiatric Morbidity Survey: Survey of Mental Health and Wellbeing.*
[6] www.nice.org.uk/guidance/cg90

developed for its brevity and acceptability for both clinician and patient. The questions are:

1. *During the last month, have you often been bothered by feeling down, depressed or hopeless?*
2. *During the last month, have you often been bothered by having little interest or pleasure in doing things?*

A positive result is an affirmative answer to either question. The screen can be used by any health professional that has contact with patients attending for reviews. NICE recommends that if there is a positive result but the professional is unable to take a full mental health history and assessment, then the patient should be referred onwards. In general practice, an example of the use of this might be a patient seeing a nurse for a hypertension review who conducts a screen and refers to a GP if the result is positive.

A meta-analysis conducted in 2017 found that the screening tool had comparable rates of sensitivity and specificity to those used in other national screening programmes.

4.2.4 Depression DSM-IV diagnostic criteria

In the case of depression NICE has recommended the use of DSM-IV over ICD-11 on the grounds that most research uses DSM-IV. DSM-IV has a marginally higher threshold for diagnosis of moderate to severe depression than does ICD-11. Nevertheless it should be recognised by clinicians that these are simply conventions to help define a very broad and heterogeneous illness. NICE also recognises that there are patients who do not meet the DSM-IV definition of depression yet have a significant functional impairment. As such, NICE has defined a subthreshold depressive category.

The DSM-IV outlines the following criteria to make a diagnosis of depression. The individual must be experiencing five or more symptoms during the same 2-week period and at least one of the symptoms should be either (1) depressed mood or (2) loss of interest or pleasure.

1. Depressed mood most of the day, nearly every day
2. Markedly diminished interest or pleasure in all, or almost all, activities most of the day, nearly every day
3. Significant weight loss when not dieting, or weight gain, or decrease or increase in appetite nearly every day
4. Psychomotor changes – agitation (physical and mental restlessness) and/or retardation (slowing down of thought and a reduction of physical movement) – observable by others, not merely subjective feelings
5. Fatigue or loss of energy nearly every day
6. Feelings of worthlessness or excessive or inappropriate guilt nearly every day
7. Diminished ability to think or concentrate, or indecisiveness, nearly every day
8. Recurrent thoughts of death, recurrent suicidal ideation without a specific plan, or a suicide attempt or a specific plan.

The DSM-IV also requires an assessment of the impact of the patient's social or occupational functioning. As such, the following criteria are also required:

1. The symptoms must cause clinically significant distress or impairment in social, occupational, or other important areas of functioning.
2. The symptoms must not be due to the direct physiological effects of a substance (e.g. drug abuse, a prescribed medication's side-effects) or a medical condition (e.g. hypothyroidism).

NICE makes it very clear in its guideline of 2009 that the diagnosis of depression should not be a matter of symptom counting. To receive a diagnosis of depression, the symptoms must cause clinically significant distress.

NICE depression definitions

Using the criteria above, NICE then defines four categories:

1. **Subthreshold depressive symptoms:** fewer than five symptoms of depression

2. **Mild depression**: few, if any, symptoms in excess of the five required to make the diagnosis, and symptoms result in only minor functional impairment

3. **Moderate depression**: symptoms of functional impairment are between 'mild' and 'severe'

4. **Severe depression**: most symptoms, and the symptoms markedly interfere with functioning; can occur with or without psychotic symptoms.

> The diagnosis of depression should not be a matter of symptom counting.

Clinicians can then use these criteria to help inform the patient's management plan.

4.2.5 Emotional and behavioural symptoms

Sadness is often stated as one of the key components of depression. However, it is extremely important to distinguish depression as a clinical diagnosis from the normal human emotion of sadness. It remains a commonly held misconception amongst the public that depression is simply on the far end of a scale of sadness. Sadness can be a perfectly rational emotion in normal human beings. Sadness can be caused by a specific event, situation or person, and it is important not to medicalise this normal state of human emotion. Whilst the DSM criteria help distinguish depression from sadness with a list of other symptoms, it is important as a clinician to understand the range of psychological and emotional symptoms that your patient may be going through which are not captured in the diagnostic criteria.

The NHS website [7] lists a group of psychological symptoms that are not all captured by the DSM criteria. These symptoms, all of which can be seen in depression, are:

- Continuous low mood or sadness
- Feeling hopeless and helpless
- Having low self-esteem
- Feeling tearful
- Feeling guilt-ridden

---

[7] www.nhs.uk/mental-health/conditions/clinical-depression/symptoms/

- Feeling irritable and intolerant of others
- Having no motivation or interest in things
- Finding it difficult to make decisions
- Not getting any enjoyment out of life
- Feeling anxious or worried
- Having suicidal thoughts or thoughts of harming yourself.

4.2.6 Physical symptoms

Depression, like anxiety, has a range of well-documented physical symptoms associated with it. One prevailing misconception in society generally is that mental health symptoms can't cause physical symptoms. Your patient may not recognise physical symptoms as related to depression.

Common physical symptoms

The following are common physical symptoms of depression:

- Moving or speaking more slowly than usual
- Changes in appetite or weight (up or down)
- Constipation
- Unexplained aches and pains
- Lack of energy
- Loss of libido
- Changes to the menstrual cycle
- Disturbed sleep
  - difficulty in getting to sleep
  - early morning waking.

Unlike anxiety, depression does not seem to cause activation of the adrenaline system. Hence patients who suffer depression without anxiety tend not to get adrenergic symptoms such as palpitations. Anxiety should be considered as a concurrent diagnosis in patients with such physical symptoms.

The precise physiological relationship between depression and physical symptoms remains unknown. However, it's likely that neurotransmitters affecting certain areas of the brain have an impact on systemic hormones such as cortisol.

Like anxiety, depression is strongly associated with the following syndromes (see *Section 4.1.5* for full details):

- Fibromyalgia – see *Section 5.2*
- Irritable bowel syndrome – see *Section 5.3*
- Chronic fatigue syndrome – see *Section 5.5*.

Unlike anxiety, depression does not seem to cause activation of the adrenaline system.

The causal relationship is not fully understood; however, it is well-documented that these conditions appear much more commonly in patients suffering with depression.

4.2.7 Patient Health Questionnaire (PHQ-9)

NICE has endorsed the PHQ-9 for measuring depression severity and responsiveness to treatment in a primary care setting. The results of the PHQ-9 may be used to make a depression diagnosis according to DSM-IV criteria. It can also be used to assess the response to treatment and as an overall marker of relapse and remission. The PHQ-9 is a subsection of the full PHQ assessment comprising 59 questions with modules on mood (PHQ-9), anxiety, alcohol, eating and somatoform disorders.

Many primary care practitioners use the PHQ-9 for diagnosis and monitoring. The patient can be asked to fill in the PHQ-9 during the consultation or between consultations. It is widely available [8] in a digital format.

The PHQ-9 asks the patient to respond to nine scenarios:

Over the last two weeks, how often have you been bothered by the following problems?

1. Little interest or pleasure in doing things
2. Feeling down, depressed or hopeless
3. Trouble falling or staying asleep or sleeping too much
4. Feeling tired or having little energy
5. Poor appetite or overeating
6. Feeling bad about yourself – or that you are a failure or have let yourself or your family down

---

[8] https://patient.info/doctor/patient-health-questionnaire-phq-9

7. Trouble concentrating on things, such as reading the newspaper or watching television
8. Moving or speaking so slowly that other people could have noticed, or the opposite – being so fidgety or restless that you have been moving around a lot more than usual
9. Thoughts that you would be better off dead or of hurting yourself in some way.

Each of these questions has an answer with an associated score:

- Not at all (score 0)
- Several days (score 1)
- More than half the days (score 2)
- Nearly every day (score 3)

The score for each of the nine answers is totalled to give the following interpretation:

- 5–10 = mild depression
- 10–18 = moderate depression
- 19–27 = severe depression

As suggested by NICE, it is strongly advisable that you do not use a 'symptom counting' score in isolation; it is important that you put this into the context of the impact of those symptoms on the patient's life. Therefore the PHQ-9 also asks a further question which does not contribute to the score but should be used for context:

If you checked off any problems, how difficult have these problems made it for you to do your work, take care of things at home, or get along with other people?

- Not difficult at all
- Somewhat difficult
- Very difficult
- Extremely difficult.

4.2.8 Suicide assessment

Suicide is the very significant mortality associated with the mental health condition of depression. The WHO estimates that every 40 seconds, somebody in the world dies by suicide and that nearly 1 million people die from this cause each year worldwide.

In the UK it remains the single biggest killer of men under the age of 50, with the most common methods being hanging, strangulation and suffocation, followed by poisoning. Men account for three-quarters of suicides.

Encouragingly, the rates have been declining over the decades – this may be due in part to better recognition and treatment. In the UK in the early 1980s the rates were 14.7 per 100 000 population, whereas in 2020 the equivalent figure was 10.1 deaths per 100 000.

A quarter of people who die from suicide have been in contact with a health professional in the previous week, and almost all within the last month. This makes the contact with the clinician a key moment to intervene.

> Every 40 seconds, somebody in the world dies by suicide.

In 2011 and 2018, NICE [9] recommended **against** the use of any specific 'risk assessment tool' for suicide. In a 2020 *Lancet* study [10] which looked at numerous such tools across the UK, they found little consistency in their use and implementation of the resultant scores. They concluded that "In line with national guidance, risk assessment should not be seen as a way to predict future behaviour and should not be used as a means of allocating treatment".

A personalised suicide assessment approach

As stated above – **do not use a suicide assessment 'tool'**.

The assessment of the individual patient will be a balance of risk. You will judge the factors increasing the risk, and those protective of the patient and therefore reducing the risk.

---

[9] www.nice.org.uk/guidance/ng105

[10] Graney, J., Hunt, I.M., Quinlivan, L. *et al.* (2020) Suicide risk assessment in UK mental health services: a national mixed-methods study." *Lancet Psychiatry*, **7(12):** 1046–1053.

Assessment advice

Asking questions about suicidal thoughts does not increase the risk of suicide and therefore these questions should be asked.

Build rapport and ask open questions, but follow up with questions that are very specific about suicide, e.g.

'Sometimes people feel that life is not worth living. Can you tell me how you feel about your own life?'

followed by

'Have you ever thought of harming yourself or trying to take your own life?'

If there is a risk of suicide, ask further questions to assess the risk, including:

- Assessing the current intent and plan:
  - is there a specific plan?
  - are there plans for others after death? suicide notes, changes to will, etc.
  - what is the lethality and frequency of plans or attempts?
- What are the specific risk factors present in the patient?
- What are the specific protective factors?

Factors which increase risk

- Previous suicide attempt or previous self-harm
- Male sex
- Unemployment
- Physical health conditions
- Disabling or painful illness, including chronic pain
- Living alone
- Being unmarried
- Alcohol and/or drug dependence
- Active severe mental illness (specifically affective disorders – particularly depression, schizophrenia, personality disorder)
- *It should be noted that studies have shown an increase in suicidal thoughts in children and young adults on initiation of certain antidepressants such as SSRIs, but research is inconclusive on whether this increases rates of actual or attempted suicide.*

Protective factors

- A strong religious faith
- Family support
- Having children at home
- A sense of responsibility for others
- Problem-solving skills.

Be mindful of sudden changes in risk factors – such as a protective factor being removed (e.g. children leaving home) or a new increase in alcohol consumption.

If a high level of risk is established, ensure safety with support through the crisis team of the local mental health service.

4.2.9 The short circuit tool for depression

As has been stated previously, the short circuit diagram is there primarily to help your patient visualise depression in the consultation room. It is not a technique to diagnose depression and whilst it simplifies the illness somewhat, it does have great use in helping your patient separate their sense of self from the illness. This can help remove the associated stigma and help the patient accept the diagnosis and engage with useful management.

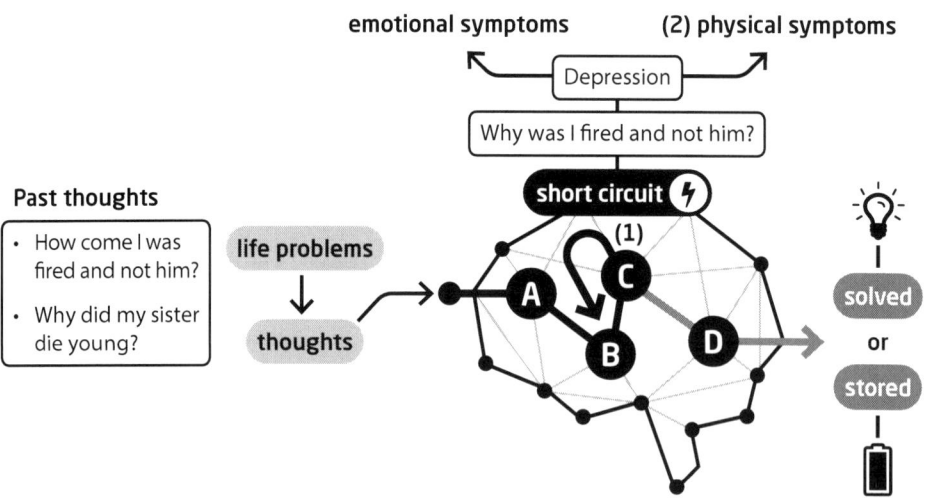

The short circuit diagram for depression looks similar to that for anxiety; however, the nature of the thoughts that become trapped in the short circuit between C and B are related to events that have already taken place. Here the thought bouncing is about the past. The past may be a distant memory from childhood or something as recent as yesterday.

I found this explanation helpful in showing patients why depression and anxiety have such different sets of symptoms associated with them. When the bouncing thought is about something that has already happened then a sense of inability to change this may ensue. This could help explain feelings such as sadness, worthlessness, emptiness and the loss of feeling of control. In contrast, the anxious patient has thought bouncing about a possible future event. In this instance the emotional demeanour is more of someone trying to prevent the future event happening, with a 'danger alarm' persistently present.

The circuit diagram also helps you describe two possible treatment targets. The first target – (1) on the diagram – aims to stop the looping, whilst the second target aims to treat physical symptoms associated with the depression. Therapies aimed at target 2 might include medicines to help with sleep or symptomatic relief from conditions such as IBS. The diagram may help to show patients that the treatment for depression itself can have a significant impact on all symptoms downstream.

4.2.10 Causes of depression

You will often hear the patient say:

'but I want to find the cause of my depression'.

This is a perfectly reasonable question which unfortunately does not have a straightforward answer. Often, a patient may be looking for a single, tangible, rational and addressable cause. Many will resist treatment until the cause is identified and rectified. Sometimes depression can be associated with biochemical anomalies such as hypothyroidism, and these should be screened for in the appropriate patients. In the interested and motivated patient you should discuss the causes as listed below; however, for a short interchange on the subject, a suggested narrative is given in *Section 2.1.4.*

It is important that you stress to your patient that a single cause is rarely identified. Specific traumatic events, for example, may trigger depression in some people and not others. Equally, many people who suffer depression will have no precipitating cause at all. The search for a cause can be frustrating and unfruitful for many, and in some cases can put them at risk of unscrupulous people or groups which purport to have the answers.

Nevertheless, the following section lists some of the known causal associations which you might find helpful when talking to individuals.

The biopsychosocial model remains the best explanation. Whilst it is not a complete or definitive answer to the question of what 'causes' depression, it helps bring together the known association into a model that tries to find a range of causal factors.

> It is important that you stress to your patient that a single cause for depression is rarely identified.

Biological causes

The biology of depression likely involves nerve cell connections, nerve cell growth, and the functioning of nerve circuits.

This notion is evidenced in the fact that whilst SSRIs cause an immediate increase in the levels of available neurotransmitter, their effect on mood can take several weeks. It may be that mood only improves as nerves grow and form new connections, a process that takes weeks and correlates well with the time of action of the SSRI. Animal studies have shown that antidepressants do spur the growth and enhanced branching of nerve cells in the hippocampus[11].

Positron emission tomography (PET), single photon emission computed tomography (SPECT) and functional magnetic reso-

---

[11] MacQueen, G. and Frodl, T. (2011) The hippocampus in major depression: evidence for the convergence of the bench and bedside in psychiatric research? *Mol Psychiatry*, **16**: 252–64.

nance imaging (fMRI) have been used to measure the distribution and density of neurotransmitter receptors in certain areas. Areas that play a significant role in mood regulation and therefore in the illness of depression are the amygdala, the thalamus and the hippocampus[12].

The amygdala is activated when a patient recalls memories, such as a frightening or stressful situation. Activity in the amygdala is higher in patients with clinically diagnosed depression. This increased activity appears to continue even after recovery from depression.

Nerve cell transmission

One of the first indications that neurotransmitters were involved in the pathogenesis of depression was the experience of reserpine – a blood pressure drug that is rarely, if ever, used now. Its mechanism of action was to reduce stores of neurotransmitter chemicals in the body's nerves. This had the effect of reducing the force of contraction of the heart, thus reducing the overall blood pressure that it produces. In addition to this effect, it also reduced stores of neurotransmitter in the brain. A large number of patients on this drug then became depressed.

Conversely, another drug, iproniazid, was initially developed as an anti-TB agent. As a side-effect it seemed to lift the mood of patients who were also depressed, and in some patients caused an abnormally elevated mood (mania). This drug was also known to increase the levels of certain neurotransmitter chemicals in the brain. Iproniazid never made it as a useful anti-TB drug but did come onto the market as one of the first ever antidepressants – only to be withdrawn later due to its other side-effects.

Whilst there is a clear link between the levels and actions of several neurotransmitters and mental health, the direct causal relationship remains uncertain.

[12] Smith, D.F. and Jakobsen, S. (2013) Molecular neurobiology of depression: PET findings on the elusive correlation with symptom severity. *Front Psychiatry*, **4**: 8.

This relationship is where the notion that depression is a 'chemical imbalance' comes from. In fact the determination of the 'quantity' of a neurotransmitter is too simplistic. Factors such as receptors' oversensitivity or insensitivity to a specific neurotransmitter may cause their response to its release to be excessive or inadequate. The neuronal growth patterns and connections are also likely to play a role.

For these complex reasons, the explanation to patients that their depression is caused by a chemical imbalance is highly unsatisfactory when used on its own.

Genetic factors

Mood is affected by dozens of genes, so the study of this factor is not easy[13]. Several genes influence the stress response, leaving certain individuals more likely to become depressed in response to stressful life situations.

Family studies have shown a propensity for depression to run in families. Bipolar disorder has the strongest link with genes – much more so than depression.

A person who has a first-degree relative who suffered major depression has an increase in risk for the condition of 1.5–3% over normal.

It would be reasonable to explain to the patient that the depression may 'run in the family'; however, the association is relatively weak.

Psychosocial factors

All people encounter stressful life events: the death of a loved one, the loss of a job, an illness, or a relationship spiralling downward. Some must cope with the early loss of a parent, violence or sexual abuse. While not everyone who faces these stresses develops a mood disorder – in fact, most do not – these stressful events likely play a role in development of depression.

Some studies have shown that people who are depressed or have dysthymia can have increased levels of corticotrophin-releasing

---

[13] Lohoff, F.W. (2010) Overview of the genetics of major depressive disorder. *Curr Psychiatry Rep*, **12**(6): 539–46.

hormone (CRH). Antidepressants are known to reduce these high CRH levels. The reduction of depressive symptoms can be associated with CRH levels returning to normal[14].

Whilst it is important to note that not all people who suffer a stressful event develop depression, it is also important to recognise that there are many people who do suffer with depression who cannot pinpoint a specific stressful trigger. The association between stressful life events and depression is clear but one does not have to be directly correlated with the other.

Trauma in early life

Studies have found that individuals experiencing trauma in childhood and early adulthood are more likely to develop depressive symptoms in later life[15]. These events can have lasting physical, as well as emotional, consequences. In particular early losses, such as the death of a parent or the withdrawal of love, may resonate throughout life, eventually expressing themselves as depression. Trauma and stress later in life can also trigger a return to depression at a much lower threshold.

Again, there is some evidence that cortisol is involved. In a study of survivors of childhood physical and sexual abuse, it was found that the stress hormones adrenocorticotrophic hormone (ACTH) and cortisol increased disproportionately when they performed stressful tasks, such as working out mathematical equations or speaking in front of an audience. Trauma during childhood may be implicated in the functioning of CRH and the hypothalamic–pituitary–adrenal axis (HPA) throughout life.

Sunlight

There is an associated rise in cases of depression during the winter months, leading to the hypothesis that sunlight and circadian

[14] Holsboer, F. and Ising, M. (2008) Central CRH system in depression and anxiety – evidence from clinical studies with CRH1 receptor antagonists. *Eur J Pharmacol*, **583**(2–3): 350–7.
[15] Negele, A., Kaufhold, J., Kallenbach, L. and Leuzinger-Bohleber, M. (2015) Childhood trauma and its relation to chronic depression in adulthood. *Depress Res Treat*, 650804.

rhythm are implicated in the pathogenesis of depression. The condition known as seasonal affective disorder (SAD) affects about 1–2% of the population, particularly women and young people. It is not entirely clear whether SAD is a form of depression or a separate entity but symptoms are similar.

A 2013 meta-analysis[16] noticed that study participants with depression also had low vitamin D levels. The same analysis found that, statistically, people with low vitamin D levels were at a much greater risk of depression. The authors stopped short of recommending vitamin D as a suitable treatment for depression. Light therapy as a treatment for depression has limited evidence.

Associated medical disease

Physical medical illnesses or medications may be implicated in up to 15% of cases of depression.

Hypothyroidism. Both hyper- and hypothyroidism can be associated with mental illness. Hypothyroidism is most associated with depression-like symptoms, and most patients with new symptoms should be screened for hypothyroidism.

Ischaemic heart disease. Up to half of MI patients report symptoms of depression. The presence of depression can be linked with slower recovery and an increased risk of further cardiovascular events.

Degenerative neurological conditions. Multiple sclerosis, Parkinson's disease, Alzheimer's disease, Huntington's chorea, stroke and dementia are strongly associated. The exact causal relationship is unclear; however, changes to the brain anatomy and changes to relative levels of neurotransmitters such as acetylcholine and dopamine are likely involved.

Population-based studies suggest that one in every three patients

---

[16] Anglin, R.E., Samaan, Z., Walter, S.D. and McDonald, S.D. (2013) Vitamin D deficiency and depression in adults: systematic review and meta-analysis. *Br J Psychiatry*, **202**: 100–7.

who develop stroke or Parkinson's disease will develop depression. Between 27% and 54% of patients with multiple sclerosis (MS) have had an episode of major depressive disorder, and 30–50% of patients with dementia have depression.

Equally, individuals suffering with depression are also more likely to develop neurological conditions, such as epilepsy, migraine, stroke, Parkinson's disease and dementia. This further complicates an already complex study of the relationship between the two.

4.2.11 Management

NICE provides substantial guidance on management of patients with depression broken down by its four categories based on the DSM-IV symptoms list given in *Section 4.2.4*, alongside the assessment of functional impairment:

- **Subthreshold depressive symptoms**: fewer than five symptoms of depression.
- **Mild depression**: few, if any, symptoms in excess of the five required to make the diagnosis, and symptoms result in only minor functional impairment.
- **Moderate depression**: symptoms of functional impairment are between 'mild' and 'severe'.
- **Severe depression**: most symptoms, and the symptoms markedly interfere with functioning; can occur with or without psychotic symptoms.

NICE stepped-care model

NICE recommends a stepped-care model in which the least intrusive, most effective intervention and most tolerable intervention is offered first before moving through the steps. Aside from the level of symptoms and functional impairment, the following factors should also be taken into account when offering a treatment:

- **Any history of depression and comorbid mental health or physical disorders**
  - the presence of this could result in starting at a higher step

- **Any past history of mood elevation (to determine if the depression may be part of bipolar disorder)**
  - if mania has been identified then an SSRI without a mood stabiliser may precipitate a manic episode and could be contraindicated – a suspicion of bipolar disease should normally prompt a secondary care referral
- **Any past experience of, and response to, treatments**
  - if a patient has had treatment failures in the past at a lower step then consider skipping this step to a more appropriate one; there is little benefit in rigidly following the steps in order if there is a recorded history of things that haven't worked in the past
- **The quality of interpersonal relationships**
  - this can influence the individual's adherence to task-oriented interventions like CBT
- **Living conditions and social isolation**
  - these can affect the patient's ability to attend courses – very isolated individuals may also not have people around them to recognise deterioration and may therefore require more intensive follow-up.

Step level	Suitable for	Treatment options
All patients	All	Risk assessment
		Education
Step 1	**Subthreshold symptoms**	Support and education
		Sleep hygiene advice
		Active monitoring
		Exercise and physical activity
Step 2	**Persistent subthreshold** depressive symptoms; **mild to moderate** depression	Low-intensity CBT
		Pharmacology
		Mindfulness-based cognitive therapy (MBCT)

Step 3	Persistent **subthreshold depressive symptoms** or **mild to moderate depression** with inadequate response to initial interventions; **moderate and severe depression**	High-intensity CBT Pharmacology Combination treatments
Step 4	**Severe and complex depression**; risk to life; severe self-neglect	Refer to secondary care Combination pharmacology

All patients

As with any other mental health treatment, before you offer the patient any form of intervention, ask yourself if the patient has understood the diagnosis and has a good concept of 'what' you are trying to treat.

If you have used the short circuit tool, you can tell them that you are trying to break the short circuit, therefore enabling all the thoughts that arise through their life problems to flow through their minds without bouncing persistently between B and C. They will still have their problems in life and they will still have a range of thoughts that naturally flow from them, but the thoughts will not be all-consuming. If the treatment is successful, they are likely to see their real personality shine through again.

Compliance will be better and therapies more likely to see success if they are fully invested in the plan, feel part of it and have been centrally involved in its inception. Starting treatment for a mental health disorder in a patient who either doesn't believe they have it or doesn't understand it, is much more likely to fail. This is where, I believe, the short circuit tool can add significantly to the patient experience.

Treatment should be offered to the patient in a stepwise fashion and in full collaboration with the patient. However, the steps should not be rigidly applied to every patient – if the patient is clearly at a higher level of disability then you should start at a higher step level. It is generally better to have a good mastery of each of these treatment modalities so that you can apply them more personally to the patient in front of you.

When offering treatments it's important to fully educate the patient about the pros and cons of each treatment. Be aware that a number of stigmas or preconceptions may exist about any type of mental health treatment, including talking therapies and medicines. Often patients may choose the wrong type of therapy based on an incorrect assumption.

Some general principles

- **Be open**, develop **trust** and have a **non-judgemental** manner at all times.
- Instil **hope and optimism** – whilst the patient's past life will not change, the illness of depression can be treated and recovery is possible.
- Be aware of **stigma**. Patients may not wish to talk about depression, it may have a negative or even offensive effect. Be mindful of this.
- Give information in an **appropriate manner** for the patient's understanding, and ensure you have informed consent.
- Be respectful of, and sensitive to **diverse cultural, ethnic and religious backgrounds** when working with people with depression, and be aware of the possible variations in the presentation of depression.

Compliance will be better and therapies more likely to see success if patients are fully invested in the plan.

Always ask people with depression directly about suicidal ideation and intent. If there is a low risk of self-harm or suicide:

- assess whether the person has adequate social support and is aware of sources of help
- arrange help appropriate to the level of risk
- advise the person to seek further help if the situation deteriorates.

If your assessment suggests a high or imminent risk – go straight to STEP 4

Step 1

Support and education

NICE Step 1 is generic advice that applies to all patients who are known or suspected to have a presentation of depression. All patients should have an appropriate assessment, support, education regarding the condition and active monitoring.

Advise a person with depression and their family or carer to be vigilant for mood changes, negativity and hopelessness, and suicidal ideation, and to contact their practitioner if concerned. This is particularly important during high-risk periods, such as starting or changing treatment and at times of increased personal stress.

Advice on sleep hygiene

- Establish regular sleep and wake times
- Avoid excess eating, smoking or drinking alcohol before sleep
- Optimise the environment for sleep (see *Section 6.2.5* for some online resources to help with this)
- Take regular physical exercise.

Active monitoring

Some people with subthreshold depressive symptoms may recover with no formal intervention – you may wish to 'watch and wait'. You should, however, ensure that you:

- discuss the presenting problem(s) and any concerns that the person may have about them
- provide information about the nature and course of depression
- arrange a further assessment, normally within 2 weeks
- make contact if the person does not attend follow-up appointments.

Exercise and physical activity

The condensed NICE guidelines (CG90, 2009) do not include this recommendation; however, it is a commonly held belief that exercise can improve symptoms of depression, and some evidence does support this notion.

Overall, the evidence indicates that group-based physical activity is effective in the treatment of subthreshold and mild depression, when compared with no physical activity controls [17]. For some people it can work as well as SSRIs in the subthreshold group;

[17] Cooney, G.M., Dwan, K., Greig, C.A. *et al.* (2013) Exercise for depression. *Cochrane Database Syst Rev,* (9)CD004366.

however, it must be stressed that exercise alone will likely be insufficient to treat patients with higher levels of depression.

Step 2

Low-intensity psychological therapies

See *Section 6.4* for a detailed consideration of CBT.

Low-intensity therapies are fundamentally a way of getting a better cost–benefit outcome for more patients. Since these methods require fewer therapists per patient, they can be deployed over a much larger patient cohort – particularly those who may not need the intensity of dedicated one-to-one sessions. Psychological therapies considered 'low-intensity' are:

- Guided self-administered CBT
  - this should be supported by a trained facilitator but the patient does much of the reading and personal reflection
  - usually consists of five to seven weekly or fortnightly face-to-face or telephone sessions, each lasting 20–30 minutes
- Psychoeducational groups
  - these are group sessions based on CBT
  - they should be conducted by trained practitioners
  - they will usually have a ratio of one therapist to about twelve participants
  - not suitable for certain forms of anxiety such as social anxiety disorder
- Computerised CBT
  - this can be used instead of face-to-face guided CBT
  - may be more accessible and convenient to some
  - evidence is currently lacking for its effectiveness.

Mindfulness-based cognitive therapy (MBCT)

Clinical results suggest that mindfulness-based therapy is a promising intervention for treating anxiety and mood problems in clinical populations [18].

---

[18] Kuyken, W., Warren, F.C., Taylor, R.S. *et al.* (2016) Efficacy of mindfulness-based cognitive therapy in prevention of depressive relapse: an individual patient data meta-analysis from randomized trials. *JAMA Psychiatry*, **73**(**6**): 565–74.

Mindfulness is recommended by NICE as a way to prevent relapse of depression symptoms. This is a mental training technique that encourages awareness of thoughts, feelings, moods and bodily sensations as they are in the present moment.

By paying attention to these thoughts and feelings right now, the patient is able to become better at spotting the build-up of difficult emotions and thoughts and can deal with them more skilfully, instead of just reacting in ways that may worsen the situation.

Drug treatments

See *Section 6.5* for a detailed consideration of pharmacological therapies.

Whilst pharmacological treatments are usually reserved for the next step, patients who present at Step 2 should be considered for drug treatment if:

- there is a past history of moderate or severe depression, or
- subthreshold depressive symptoms or mild depression have been present for a long period (typically at least 2 years), or
- there are subthreshold depressive symptoms or mild depression that persist after other interventions have failed.

Step 3

High-intensity CBT

High-intensity differs from low-intensity in that this is usually done in a one-to-one setting with a trained therapist. It is based on the principles of CBT. The therapist will have regular supervision to monitor fidelity to the treatment mode, will use routine outcome measures and ensure that the patient is involved in reviewing the efficacy of the treatment.

Unlike the low-intensity version, here the patient will normally have 12–15 weekly sessions (fewer if the person recovers sooner; more if clinically required), each lasting one hour.

Pharmacological treatments

NICE recommends that antidepressants are not routinely used to treat persistent subthreshold depressive symptoms or mild depression; however, even in this group, there may be a place if:

- there is a past history of moderate or severe depression
- subthreshold depressive symptoms have persisted for a long period
- subthreshold depressive symptoms persist after other interventions have been tried.

Before starting any antidepressant medication it is fundamentally important to explore the patient's beliefs, understanding and concerns around these drugs.

Drug treatment options – for antidepressant effect

- SSRIs
  - these will normally be the first line in almost all patients
- SNRIs
  - second-line for those not responsive to SSRIs
- Tricyclics
  - second- or third-line – low-dose TCAs will not have an antidepressant effect
- Mirtazapine
  - usually second-line – has benefits in helping sleep
- Monoamine oxidase inhibitors (MAOIs)
  - rarely used, although newer reversible agents are now available; not started in primary care but may be in secondary care
- Antipsychotics
  - for depression with psychosis; generally reserved for initiation in secondary care.

When an antidepressant is to be prescribed, it should normally be an SSRI in a generic form, because SSRIs are equally effective as other antidepressants and have a favourable risk–benefit ratio.

Drug treatment options – agitation/sleep disturbance

- Antihistamines
  - available over the counter; generally safe, not addictive but can produce tolerance effects
- Benzodiazepines
  - very addictive – recommended for short-term use only
- Z-drugs (e.g. zopiclone)
  - addictive – recommended for short-term use only.

Drug combinations and augmentation

Some antidepressant drugs can be combined and used as augmenters. This strategy usually requires the input of secondary care services, but some primary care practitioners will use these strategies if they are comfortable and competent.

NICE makes it clear that no class of antidepressant should be augmented with:

- a benzodiazepine for more than 2 weeks (significant risk of dependence)
- buspirone, carbamazepine, lamotrigine or valproate (insufficient evidence)
- pindolol or thyroid hormones (inconsistent evidence of effectiveness).

Some drugs are used in combination such as SSRI or SNRI with:

- lithium
- an antipsychotic (e.g. quetiapine)
- another antidepressant, such as mirtazapine.

Be aware that there may be a diminishing return and that side-effects may increase.

Step 4

Referral to specialist mental health services should normally be for people with depression who are at significant risk of self-harm, have psychotic symptoms, require complex multiprofessional care, or where an expert opinion on treatment and management is needed.

Crisis resolution teams

Crisis teams, or crisis resolution and home treatment teams, are ubiquitously commissioned across the UK. They are there to provide support when a patient is in an acute state of distress and might otherwise need to go to a hospital. Indications for referral to crisis resolution include (but are not limited to):

- patients who are in a current state of high risk of suicide
- patients going through acute relapse of psychotic symptoms
- patients who are at high risk of acute hospital admission as a result of a mental health issue.

If after a personal assessment of a patient's risk of suicide you find that they are at high risk, you should immediately refer them to the local crisis home resolution team. You should make yourself aware of their referral portal locally (this is usually a phone number).

The crisis resolution team can:

- visit the patient in their home or elsewhere in the community, for example at a crisis house or day centre
- assess the patient's needs and offer support including:
  - assistance with self-help strategies
  - administering (and usually prescribing) medication
  - providing practical help, for example with money, housing or childcare arrangements
  - care planning and prevention for any future crisis
- liaise with consultant psychiatrists in the case of escalation of medical treatment or admission to a mental health unit
- follow the patient up on a regular basis as appropriate (this could be daily) until the crisis state is resolved.

Crisis resolution teams also work with acute hospital Trusts where patients attend the Emergency Department with a mental health issue.

Secondary care referrals

The exact choice of who to refer to a secondary care service and when will, of course, depend on the individual clinician and their patient. Factors influencing this might include the primary care clinician's own level of expertise and comfort with a higher level of pathology. Nevertheless, these features should normally trigger a referral into secondary care:

- Any patient with features of psychosis (delusional thought disorders and auditory hallucinations)
- Patients with any concurrent severe mental illness (such as bipolar or schizophrenia)
- Patients who are at significant risk of self-harm
- Patients who require complex care across multiple agencies
- Patients where treatments have failed across multiple steps or who require multidrug augmentation therapies (see *Section 6.4.13*).

4.2.12 Depression in children and young people

In 2019, NICE published guidance specifically around the management of depression for children and young people, aimed at those aged 5–18 years[19].

A detailed review of the care of children with depression is outside the scope of this book; however, the following are useful points from the 2019 NICE guidance.

General principles

Children from the age of 5 can suffer with depression, anxiety and other mental illnesses – you should be aware and alert to recognising this. Numbers of diagnosis in young people have risen sharply in recent years and it is hypothesised that this is due to greater detection. It is estimated that the prevalence of depression in teenagers is about 6% and anxiety just over 10%.

You should engage with both the child and the family, and where possible and appropriate speak to the child on their own. In

---

[19] NICE (2019) *Depression in children and young people: identification and management*. NICE guideline [NG134].

addition to the usual considerations in a mental health history, you should always ask the patient and their parents or carers directly about:

- the child or young person's alcohol and drug use
- any experience of being bullied or abused
- self-harm and ideas about suicide.

Making a diagnosis

A definitive diagnosis of anything above mild depression in children from the age of 5 should be made in a Child and Adolescent Mental Health Services (CAMHS) service. From primary care, consider referral if the child meets the following criteria:

- Depression with two or more other risk factors for depression
- Depression where one or more family members (parents or children) have multiple-risk histories for depression
- Mild depression in those who have not responded to interventions in tier 1 after 2–3 months
- Moderate or severe depression (including psychotic depression)
- Signs of a recurrence of depression in those who have recovered from previous moderate or severe depression
- Unexplained self-neglect of at least one month's duration that could be harmful to their physical health
- Active suicidal ideas or plans
- Referral requested by a young person or their parents or carers.

Treatment considerations

The NICE guidance breaks down treatment options by age of child and severity of illness.

	5–11-year-olds	12–18-year-olds
Mild depression (including dysthymia)	**Watchful waiting** (review in 2 weeks) **Digital** or **group CBT** **Interpersonal therapy** **Group non-directive supportive therapy** If the child has reached a level of development and their needs are not met • **individual CBT** • or **attachment-based family therapy** NICE does not recommend antidepressant medicines in this group This group can normally be managed in primary/community care; if they do not respond to interventions, *refer through CAMHS*	
Moderate to severe depression	Family-based IPT Psychodynamic psychotherapy Individual CBT	Individual CBT for at least 3 months SSRI + CBT (use fluoxetine)

Mood and Feelings Questionnaire

The Mood and Feelings Questionnaire (MFQ) is available in a long and short version. Each of these has a child self-report version and a parent or carer report version which is completed by the child and parent, respectively. Developed in the 1980s, it has been extensively tested and is approved by NICE as a relevant and appropriate marker of the extent of depression severity. It can be used as a guide for progress of treatment. It can be found widely online [20].

Specific child psychological therapies

Interpersonal therapy and family interpersonal therapy
Interpersonal psychotherapy (IPT) for young people with depression looks at the relationships around the young person. It helps them to make sense of the difficulties they are experiencing and

---

[20] https://devepi.duhs.duke.edu/measures/the-mood-and-feelings-questionnaire-mfq/

to understand how their relationships with other people contribute to how they feel. It is generally considered a short-term treatment that is effective in treating depression in children.

Depression often occurs in the context of an individual's relationships, and this can be independent of any other causes rooted in biology or genetics. Interpersonal therapy effectively aims to break the cycle of depression affecting relationships and which then in turn further affect mood.

Attachment-based family therapy

This is a type of family therapy in which the therapist aims to help a parent and a child repair ruptures in their relationship and work to develop or rebuild an emotionally secure relationship. In this respect is has a very similar foundation to interpersonal therapy; however, it draws much more on the principles of attachment theory. This form of therapy has empirical evidence supporting it as an effective treatment for adolescents experiencing suicidal ideation or depression.

Using SSRIs in children and young people

SSRIs can be safely used in children and adolescents over the age of 12 years. However, NICE has made the following recommendations:

- SSRIs should not be used for mild depression
- If an SSRI is to be used, the child should have had an assessment and diagnosis by a child and adolescent psychiatrist
- Do not offer them except in combination with a concurrent psychological therapy
- You should carefully monitor for adverse drug reactions and review general mental state – the suggestion is **weekly for the first 4 weeks of treatment**
  - *in particular, closely monitor for the appearance of suicidal behaviour, self-harm or hostility at the beginning of treatment; the initial phase has, in some studies, been associated with a rise in these symptoms*
- Use fluoxetine as this is the only antidepressant for which clinical trial evidence shows that the benefits outweigh the risks

- Start at a dose of 10mg and increase to 20mg only if clinically needed. Evidence for efficacy of higher doses is limited.

In some case sertraline or citalopram can be used but these are strictly second-line. NICE states that paroxetine, SNRIs and TCAs should not be used for the treatment of depression in children and young people.

4.2.13 Course and prognosis

Roughly half of all cases of mild to moderate depression will resolve slowly over time. In one meta-analysis, 25% of patients with mild to moderate depression saw their symptoms resolve within 3 months, and about 50% of patients saw symptoms resolve within 12 months[21]. This clearly indicates that the condition can be self-limiting, but this could take a long time and improve in only 25–50% of patients.

For those patients that reach the criteria of moderate to severe depression, up to 80% will have at least one more episode in their lifetime. The average number of relapses will be between four and five, with some patients experiencing many more. Virtually all patients with psychotic symptoms relapse.

In light of this, depression, certainly for patients who have had more than one episode, should be considered a chronic remitting and relapsing condition. For these patients a long-term (even lifelong) treatment with an antidepressant such as an SSRI, as a prophylactic measure, should be considered. A number of studies have concluded that the increase in usage of SSRIs overall in the population has resulted in a drop in the levels of suicide – e.g. in Sweden in the 1990s, a threefold increase in SSRI use resulted in a 25% drop in suicide rates[22].

[21] Whiteford, H.A., Harris, M.G., McKeon, G. *et al.* (2012) Estimating remission from untreated major depression: a systematic review and meta-analysis. *Psychological Medicine*, **43(8):** 1569–1585.
[22] Isacsson, G., Bergman, U. and Rich, C.L. (1996) Epidemiological data suggest antidepressants reduce suicide risk among depressives. *J Affect Disord*, **41:** 1–8.

A poorer outcome is predicted in patients with the following features:

- Those who receive non-standard treatment
- Severe initial symptoms including psychosis
- Early age of onset
- Multiple previous episodes
- Incomplete recovery after one year of treatment
- Pre-existing severe mental or medical disorder
- High levels of family dysfunction.

It should also be noted that life expectancy for patients suffering from depression is lower than in the general population. This is in part due to the mortality associated with suicide but also due to higher prevalence of other medical illness such as ischaemic heart disease.

4.3 Focus on OCD

> **What you'll learn in this section**
>
> This section describes the classification, epidemiology, diagnosis and treatment of OCD.
>
> **How this helps**
>
> OCD is a commonly seen illness and clinicians should have a good grasp of its diagnosis and management.

Obsessive–compulsive disorder (OCD) is a commonly seen mental health disorder in primary care. The patient has certain thoughts repeatedly (obsessions) or feels the need to perform certain routines repeatedly (compulsions). These obsessions and compulsions generate distress and often have a significant effect on the general functioning of the individual, including impacts on their social life and work. Common compulsions include hand washing, counting of things, and repeated checking (e.g. to ascertain whether a door is locked).

Whilst some of these symptoms are present in many 'normal' people, those with OCD pathology will spend several hours per day dedicated to addressing and calming the compulsions. It is the cause of suicide in some individuals.

4.3.1 Classifications of OCD

In ICD-10, OCD sat under the category of 'Neurotic, stress-related and somatoform disorders', alongside other anxiety-related disorders. This was broken down further into 'Predominantly obsessional thoughts or ruminations', 'Predominantly compulsive acts' or 'Mixed obsessional thoughts and acts'. However, significant changes were made in ICD-11.

ICD-11 categorisation

In ICD-11 (released in 2018 as a preliminary version), obsessive–compulsive disorder sits in its own category of *Obsessive-*

Compulsive or Related Disorders and within that, the following subcategories exist:

- Obsessive–compulsive disorder
- Body dysmorphic disorder
- Olfactory reference disorder
- Hypochondriasis
- Hoarding disorder
- Body-focused repetitive behaviour disorders
- Substance-induced obsessive–compulsive or related disorders
- Secondary obsessive–compulsive or related syndrome
- Other specified obsessive–compulsive or related disorders
- Obsessive–compulsive or related disorders, unspecified.

4.3.2 Epidemiology

Obsessive–compulsive disorder affects about 2.3% of people at some point in their life, with the yearly rate about 1.2%. Symptoms usually begin before the age of 35 and half of sufferers develop symptoms before age 20. Males and females are affected equally.

> Most patients have had symptoms of OCD for 5 to 10 years before presentation.

4.3.3 Screening tools and presentation

NICE has, in the past, recommended that for people known to be at higher risk of OCD (such as individuals with other mental health conditions or substance misuse), healthcare professionals should routinely consider and explore the possibility of OCD by asking direct questions such as:

- 'Do you wash or clean a lot?'
- 'Do you check things a lot?'
- 'Is there any thought that keeps bothering you that you would like to get rid of but cannot?'
- 'Do your daily activities take a long time to finish?'
- 'Are you concerned about putting things in a special order or are you very upset by mess?'
- 'Do these problems trouble you?'

These may not be very specific screening questions, however. Many people have harmless personal preferences or personality quirks which mean they prefer a cleaner environment or like to have a shiny car, therefore wax it many times. The key difference with OCD is that these symptoms become extremely intrusive and disruptive and take up a large proportion of the patient's day and thought processes, despite them fighting the urge to perform obsessive–compulsive tasks.

You should also be vigilant for the physical symptoms and signs associated with some of the subsets of OCD, e.g.:

- Body dysmorphic disorder
  - repeated cosmetic procedures with little satisfaction
  - consultations about minor skin flaws and worries about body shape
- Trichotillomania
  - noticeable hair loss, such as shortened hair or thinned or bald areas on the scalp or other areas of the body, including sparse or missing eyelashes or eyebrows
- Excoriation (skin picking) disorder
  - developing recurring skin lesions or open wounds due to picking
  - moles, freckles, spots that have been picked to try to 'smooth' or 'perfect' them.

4.3.4 OCD symptoms and diagnosis

The term OCD is often misused in medicine and by society at large. Like many other mental health disorders, it can exist on a spectrum from mild to extremely dysfunctional. You may be asked, as a primary care clinician, if something 'sounds' like OCD. The three criteria detailed below are present in those with OCD as a mental health disorder and are not found in those people who simply have a quirky or unusual habit or desire for doing certain tasks. The formal diagnosis of OCD is a clinical one and is sometimes done in primary care, where the clinician feels confident and comfortable

> Symptoms of OCD become extremely intrusive and disruptive and take up a large proportion of the patient's day and thought processes.

with this, or is done formally in secondary care. It often needs more than a single session to achieve a confident diagnosis.

The diagnosis is usually based on the 'clinically significant' obsession and compulsion **and** the time spent per day on these tasks.

Clinically significant obsession

These are obsessions that are recurrent and persistent thoughts, impulses or images that are experienced as intrusive and that cause marked anxiety or distress. These lie outside the normal range of worries about conventional problems (be careful, as this element can be subjective). The patient will be trying to ignore or suppress such obsessions, or to neutralise them with some other thought or action. They will almost always recognise the obsessive thought as irrational.

Clinically significant compulsion

Compulsions are clinically significant when the patient feels driven to perform them in response to an obsession and in accordance with rules that must be applied rigidly. The key difference between a clinically significant compulsion and a person with a quirk of personality is that the OCD sufferer **must** perform these actions to avoid significant psychological distress. Often the actions are done to prevent or reduce distress or perceived negative outcome, rather than to achieve some logical or practical aim. At some point during the course of the disorder, the individual **will** realise that the obsessions or compulsions are unreasonable or excessive.

Time-consumption

The obsessions or compulsions must be time-consuming (taking up more than one hour per day) or cause impairment in social, occupational or school functioning.

The presence of these three items is a good indicator of the presence of the pathology of OCD.

Yale-Brown OCD Scale

The Yale–Brown Obsessive Compulsive Scale (Y-BOCS) is a test to rate the severity of OCD symptoms. There is also a corresponding children's version. The Y-BOCS is a 10-item observer-rating scale. A total score of ≥16 is considered to be indicative of clinically significant OCD. The Y-BOCS severity scale has an associated symptom checklist of fifteen categories of obsessions and compulsions. The full test can be found online [23]. It is completed by the patient themselves and takes about 10 minutes. It is often considered the gold standard for measuring the severity of a person's OCD. It can also be used to monitor progress of therapy and intervention.

4.3.5 The short circuit tool for OCD

The short circuit diagram is there to help your patient visualise the illness in the consultation room. It is not a technique to diagnose. It simplifies the illness somewhat but it does have great use in helping your patient separate their sense of self from the illness. This can help remove the associated stigma and help the patient accept the diagnosis and engage with useful management.

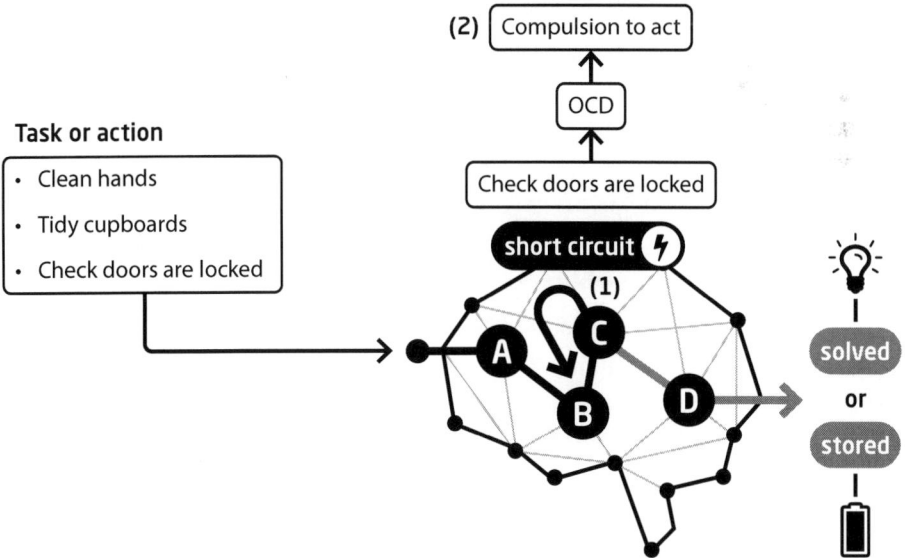

---

[23] https://iocdf.org/wp-content/uploads/2014/08/Assessment-Tools.pdf

The short circuit diagram for OCD looks similar to that for anxiety or depression; however, the nature of the thoughts that become trapped in the short circuit between C and B are related to tasks and actions rather than events or memories.

This analogy can be helpful in showing patients the trapped thought cycle. The list of actions or tasks to be completed are not, in themselves, unusual or uncommon, but the pathology lies in the fact that they are trapped by a short circuit. This can help explain the excess and distressing thoughts – or obsessions about a particular task. This then leads to the compulsion to act on that thought, which gives the patient some temporary relief from the cycling, but since the short circuit still exists, the bouncing restarts. This gives the patient the recurrent cycle of obsession followed by compulsion.

Whilst the thought bounces continuously, the patient can get many distressing emotional and physical symptoms which can mimic those found in anxiety or depression.

The circuit diagram also helps you describe two possible treatment targets. The first target – (1) on the diagram – aims to stop the looping, whilst the second target aims to stop the acting out of the compulsions and can address more 'downstream' physical symptoms such as sleeplessness and agitation.

4.3.6 Causes of OCD

The cause of OCD remains unknown. However, environmental, genetic, neurochemical, anatomical and drug factors could play a role. Risk factors include a history of child abuse or the presence of multiple stress-inducing events.

Neurochemical studies, particularly on the action of SSRIs, SNRIs and antipsychotics, suggest a significant role for both serotonin and dopamine. Neuroimaging studies have shown that both the orbitofrontal cortex and basal ganglia are likely involved in the pathological process[24].

---

[24] Parmar, A. and Sarkar, S. (2016) Neuroimaging studies in obsessive compulsive disorder: a narrative review. *Indian J Psychol Med*, **38**(**5**): 386–94.

Drug-induced

Drug-induced OCD generally assumes that the patient did not have OCD before the ingestion of the drugs. OCD symptoms are associated with the acute ingestion of stimulant drugs such as cocaine or amphetamines and their chronic abuse. Atypical antipsychotics such as olanzapine have also been shown to induce OCD in patients who did not have this prior to starting those drugs.

Genetics

There is some evidence of a genetic component. Identical twins are more often affected than non-identical twins raised in the same family and environment. Individuals with OCD are more likely to have first-degree family members exhibiting the same disorder. The familial link is stronger with OCD which develops in childhood compared to OCD which develops in adulthood[25].

> Risk factors of OCD include a history of child abuse or the presence of multiple stress-inducing events.

4.3.7 Management

NICE guidelines[26] were last published in full in 2005; however, there have been several evidence updates since.

General principles of care

NICE states that "People with OCD are often ashamed and embarrassed by their condition and may find it very difficult to discuss their symptoms with healthcare professionals, friends, family or carers... Healthcare professionals should help patients, and their families or carers where appropriate, to understand the involuntary nature of the symptoms."

It is therefore important that you start any therapeutic journey with the patient by explaining that the condition is not a part of their inherent personality. You should convey that the symptoms

---

[25] Kim, S.J. and Kim, C.H. (2006) The genetic studies of obsessive-compulsive disorder and its future directions. *Yonsei Med J*, **47**(4): 443–54.

[26] NICE (2005) *Obsessive-compulsive disorder and body dysmorphic disorder: treatment.* Clinical guideline [CG31].

they are getting are due to an underlying pathology, no different to any other physical pathology, and that by attempting to treat the underlying pathology, they may find relief.

The short circuit tool can be invaluable in achieving this.

Mild illness: Patients with mild illness, defined by NICE as mild functional impairment, should be offered low-intensity CBT. Specifically for OCD, a CBT technique called ERP (exposure and response prevention therapy) is often used – see below.

Moderate illness: Patients with moderate functional impairment or those with mild functional impairment who are unable to engage in low-intensity CBT or for whom low intensity treatment has proved to be inadequate should be offered either high-intensity CBT (including ERP) or SSRI.

Severe illness: Patients with severe functional impairment or those with moderate functional impairment who have failed to respond to an SSRI or high-intensity CBT should be offered a combination of both SSRI and high-intensity CBT (including ERP). Secondary care referral should be considered.

Exposure and response prevention for OCD
See *Section 6.4* for a detailed consideration of CBT.

Exposure and response prevention (ERP) is a specific technique used in CBT which involves teaching the person to deliberately come into contact with the situations that trigger the obsessive thoughts and fears ('exposure') without carrying out the usual compulsive acts associated with the obsession ('response prevention'). This gradually enables the patient to learn to tolerate the discomfort and anxiety associated with not performing the ritualistic behaviour.

An example of graduated exposure might include a patient getting 'closer' to being in a 'contaminated' area such as a bus. The patient may start off by holding a tissue that has been next to a bag that belongs to a person who regularly uses a bus. Over time the patient gets closer to direct contact with the anxiety-producing scenario or object.

The 'response prevention' component is the deliberate withholding of the normal response – which in this example would be washing hands.

Another example might be leaving the house and checking the lock only once (exposure) without going back and checking again (response prevention). The theory is that the patient quickly adjusts to the anxiety-producing situation. The relative levels of exposure can increase under the guidance of a therapist if in a high-intensity regime, or self-managed in a low-intensity, self-directed regime.

ERP does have a reasonably strong evidence base, although, like many CBT studies, many suffer from lack of blinding and some have been criticised for being of poor quality. A 2007 Cochrane review[27] found that psychological interventions derived from CBT models were more effective than treatment as usual consisting of no treatment, waiting list or non-CBT interventions.

Psychotherapeutic intervention such as ERP-based CBT, in combination with medication, is likely to be more efficacious than either option alone.

Pharmacology

See *Section 6.5* for a detailed consideration of pharmacological therapies.

SSRIs

SSRIs are the clear mainstay of OCD treatment. More than twenty blinded, placebo-controlled studies have firmly established the efficacy of SSRI monotherapy in OCD. Proven efficacy and a benign side-effect profile have firmly established SSRIs as first-line.

Some studies have suggested that the dose of SSRI needs to be higher in OCD than the equivalent for depression and can take longer to achieve their maximal effect. The patient should be counselled on this before starting. NICE, however, does not advise a specific SSRI dose; moreover, it suggests a gradual tapered

[27] Gava, I., Barbui, C., Aguglia, E. et al. (2007) Psychological treatments versus treatment as usual for obsessive compulsive disorder (OCD). *Cochrane Database of Systematic Reviews*, Issue 2. Art. No.: CD005333.

increase as per response and manufacturer's guidelines. Some psychiatrists will use SSRI beyond their normal highest dose range, although this is ill-advised in primary care.

There is little evidence to suggest that one SSRI is superior to another.

SNRIs

It has been suggested that SNRIs should have an effect in OCD; however, this has not been backed up by any solid evidence base. Therefore, they cannot be recommended for OCD. NICE suggests that they are not used.

Clomipramine

The tricyclic antidepressant clomipramine has been shown to be beneficial in patients with OCD. Clomipramine may even be more efficacious than the SSRIs; however, it is associated with significantly more side-effects. Clomipramine is not generally considered a first-line agent but NICE does include it in guidelines as an alternative if SSRI monotherapy fails.

NICE is clear that other than clomipramine, no other tricyclic antidepressant medication is indicated for OCD.

Antipsychotics

Whilst evidence is poor, for some very refractory patients, an augmentation strategy of an atypical antipsychotic with an SSRI or clomipramine may be tried. This would be strictly under secondary care only.

4.3.8 Course and prognosis

OCD rarely, if ever, resolves spontaneously. Most patients have had symptoms for 5 to 10 years before presentation. For most patients, OCD will be a chronic disease with a remitting and relapsing pattern. Patients diagnosed in childhood will have the disorder into adulthood in approximately 40% of cases, whilst 40% will reach a position of complete remission. They will, however, have a significantly higher risk than the general population of diagnosis in later life.

Chapter 5

Physical illness with mental health connections

5.1 Focus on physical symptoms

What you'll learn in this section

Physical symptoms are common in mental health disorders. Intuitively, it can be difficult to see how a mental health problem can produce physical symptoms. This section describes how this is possible and indeed common.

How this helps:

By providing the patient with an understanding of how mental health and physical symptoms are interlinked, you help them rationalise their condition.

Personally, I think it is a great shame that over the history of medical and social science we have kept mental and physical health as separate entities. In reality, on a physiological and pathological level mental and physical health are fundamentally intertwined. Mental illness can have clear and distinct physical manifestations and any physical chronic illness can have mental health manifestations. The fact that, for many laypeople, these two entities are separate makes it difficult for people to understand and rationalise how they can be linked. When a patient is having physical symptoms it can be very difficult for them to understand that an illness like depression or anxiety may be the underlying driver. However, through a skilful consultation it is perfectly possible to help the average intelligent layperson decipher the link. When patients can rationalise their symptoms it makes it easier for them to accept and understand treatments which they may otherwise reject.

In fact, the sensations produced by the illness of depression or anxiety are as vast as they are strange. Common physical symptoms of anxiety can be palpitations, chest pain, shortness of breath or numbness in the fingertips. However, there are cases of patients becoming blind in a portion of their vision or losing their voice entirely. Specialists in ENT medicine may find no physical abnormality at the voice box, but the symptoms of being unable to properly speak remain in psychogenic dysphonia. Many of these patients are told in these scenarios that there is 'nothing wrong' with them. This is one of the most frustrating things for me to hear said about a patient's symptoms and it is sadly a phrase all too often used by medics as well as the public. A more accurate term would be that there is 'nothing anatomically wrong with the larynx'. If there was indeed 'nothing wrong at all', then the patient would not have a lost voice.

In this chapter we will discuss the physiological links between mental and physical health. There will also be specific sections on the following common conditions which have a clear association with mental illness:

- Fibromyalgia (*Section 5.2*)
- Irritable bowel syndrome (*Section 5.3*)
- Chronic pain (*Section 5.4*)
- Chronic fatigue syndrome (*Section 5.5*).

5.1.1 A direct hormonal mechanism

Anxiety, as described in *Section 4.2*, can elicit the adrenergic 'flight or fight' response.

To summarise:

Adrenaline and cortisol, along with other hormones, are released once the danger alarms are triggered. This stimulation of beta-adrenergic receptors increases the pulse and blood pressure, relaxes smooth muscles in the lungs, breaks down glycogen and diverts blood from non-essential organs. This produces the typical set of adrenergic 'panic' symptoms of palpitations, tension in the muscles, increased sweat production, sensation of shortness of breath and tingling in the fingers.

These are all fundamental physical symptoms and the patient may well come to the seemingly logical conclusion that these are caused by a defect in the heart or lungs. This then has a positive feedback loop in the cognitive symptoms of anxiety – known as secondary anxiety.

5.1.2 Another mechanism for somatic symptoms

Whilst the symptoms associated with anxiety and adrenaline may have a relatively straightforward mechanism, mental illness can result in a range of other sensory symptoms which are very difficult, at first glance, to associate with a mental health diagnosis. These can include sensory changes in the limbs, bowel symptoms, pain and fatigue, amongst others.

The pathways of sensation

I will start with the physiological explanation, followed by something which may be easier to explain to the patient. The following will serve as a useful recap of basic peripheral and central nerve physiology, but also highlight the often overlooked role of the limbic system in the genesis of sensation in the human mind.

Consider this basic nerve diagram, showing nerve impulses moving from a limb to the sensory cortex.

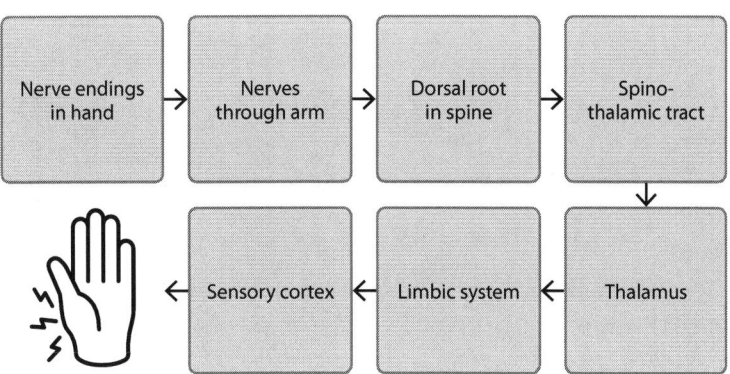

The patient, from a sensory point of view, can feel touch, pain, paraesthesia, anaesthesia, hot or cold, etc. For any sensation to be physically perceived, it needs to stimulate the sensory cortex of the brain. Stroke patients who have infarcts in this cortex will get hemiplegic sensory loss and will be unable to sense pain despite any stimulus to the relevant body part.

The pain pathway from the hand, as in the diagram above, starts with nerve endings in the organ itself. Different receptors exist for different types of stimulus, namely for heat/cold sensation, for light touch and for pain. If the hand comes into contact with a sudden stimulus, such as a sharp knife, the nerve ending in this area of the body will fire off and the brain will sense pain. This is the most common, well-recognised, and fairly intuitive cause of pain.

Following the whole pathway it is clear to see how pathology at any point can produce the same symptoms.

Patient symptom: Pain/sensation change in the hand

Site of pathology	Example of pathology	Symptom felt
Hand (nerve endings in skin)	Burn to skin	Pain/sensory changes in hand
Nerves through arm	Peripheral neuropathy, e.g. diabetes Laceration to nerves from hand, e.g. amputation	Pain/sensory changes in hand
Dorsal root in spine and spinothalamic tract	Spinal injury (cervical spine) Disc prolapse (cervical spine)	Pain/sensory changes in hand
Thalamus	Traumatic brain injury CVA	Pain/sensory changes in hand
Limbic system	*Depression* *Anxiety*	*Pain/sensory changes in hand*
Sensory cortex	CVA/MS	Pain/sensory changes in hand

When the signal reaches the brain, it has to convert these into a meaningful sensation, which may lead to a thought or action. It remains unknown how this happens.

The nerve fibres pass through several areas of the brain – these being the thalamus, which acts as a hub – bringing in information from all senses of the body, including vision, hearing, touch, smell and taste. The thalamus starts to process the vast information that it receives every second to make it meaningful to the higher centres of the brain. This information then passes through the limbic system before reaching the neocortex.

The limbic system, rather than being an individual structure, is actually a set of areas which appear symmetrically on both sides of the brain and are believed to be responsible for memory, emotion, recognition and learning. After passing through the limbic system, the signal reaches the neocortex and now the myriad of electrical signals form a sensation, thought, idea or feeling in some conscious way. This is where pain becomes a palpable entity. This is also where a person's individuality is expressed. We are the person we are due to our neocortex. It is the seat of personality and uniqueness.

So, there is a final common pathway for almost all sensory input: the limbic system and then the neocortex. And it is this area that is strongly affected by depression and anxiety. At other points in the nerve's tract, from the limb to the neocortex, it may simply be physically pinched or distorted and these disturbances will produce the sensation of pain in the relevant area. However, at the level of the limbic system, the interference is far more complex.

Depression, anxiety and other mental health conditions are strongly associated with depletion or disturbance of the neurotransmitters serotonin and dopamine. The limbic system is heavily reliant on these chemicals. Illness like this can cause a myriad of disturbances at this level in the brain. Since this process is so involved in sensory function of the body, depression can therefore cause a disturbance in almost any sensation. It is for this reason that interference at the limbic system, by illnesses such as depression, can have the effect of causing pain. The effect may not be the whole cause of the painful sensation but it may be altering the signal – making the pain more intense, for example. In fact, almost any physical symptom that the brain can perceive can be affected by disorders of the mind and mood.

Explaining this to the patient

Many people would be much happier to believe there was a problem with the organ or limb than for there to be an illness of the mind. If the problem is 'in the mind' then surely they can just snap out of it, surely it's their own doing and surely it isn't a 'real' illness? For many people, the notion that their physical symptoms are caused by a mental illness is akin to saying that they don't really have the symptoms – that they are making it up and it's 'all in their head'. It can be perceived as offensive to some patients to make this suggestion. It should therefore be done with care. Giving the patient a clear logical and scientific explanation will go a long way to easing any resistance to the exploration of mental health causing physical symptoms.

It should be noted by all involved in the care of the patient that the physical sensations caused by a mental illness are identical to the organic equivalent. The pain of fibromyalgia is real, palpable and indistinguishable from pain caused by an inflammatory arthritis in the perception of the patient.

It would be difficult to go through human physiology in any real detail in a 10-minute consultation. However, there are a number of quick analogies that you can give. Fundamentally you are trying to get the point across that a mental health condition can produce a range of seemingly unconnected and difficult to rationalise physical symptoms. In many cases, without the understanding of this connection, patients with somatic symptoms can become frustrated and need repeated consultations from a range of different specialties or a battery of tests which come back negative. This can lead to the 'medically unexplained symptoms' situation where the doctor is unable to give the patient a clear, coherent explanation for their symptoms. In some of these cases, the mental health element remains completely unexplored. In some cases, the treatment of the mental health condition can result in dramatic improvement in the physical symptoms. In other cases, pain-relieving drugs such as morphine can be dramatically reduced through appropriate treatment of the mental health condition. Where this is the case, it is very important to help the patient understand the link, as the benefit to them could be huge.

Here are a few ways in which you could try to explain things to your patient:

Consultation tip - the light bulb

In explaining the phenomenon, it might be useful to compare this to an electrical circuit. Consider the circuit that exists to turn on the light bulb in a table lamp. We know it works because the light comes on when we flip the switch. But what about when something goes wrong? Show your patient the diagram below.

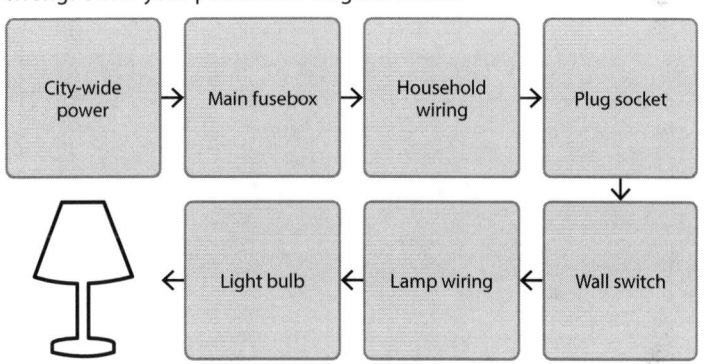

We only really have one symptom that can occur… that the light fails to come on. If the light does not come on, we know that there is something wrong. However, what we don't know is where the fault is. This is because almost any fault along the necessary path to lighting the bulb will produce the exact same symptom, i.e. no light. The fault could be that the bulb itself is damaged. It may be the wiring to the bulb that is the problem; it could be a fault in the switch; or it could be an electric fault in the house. In fact, even a power cut to the whole city would result in exactly the same symptom. Without further investigation, we cannot know what the cause of the bulb failure is. In this scenario, we have a relatively complex system at play to keep the bulb on, but a very simple and limited set of symptoms that the system can produce when something along the way goes wrong.

Most people can clearly relate to the notion that just because the light does not come on, it doesn't mean the issue is with the light bulb – the true 'pathology' could be anywhere in the circuit. In this analogy, you can say the limbic system is similarly part of the circuit and therefore mental illness can cause the same symptoms.

Consultation tip - nervous vomiting

This is a very good relatable example of mental stress causing a physical illness and a quick simple analogy that I personally use a lot.

Many of us have known people to feel sick or even actually vomit before a big stressful occasion; a driving test for example. The feeling is real. The affected individual is not making it up – they feel sick in exactly the same way as any other person with nausea. However, a thorough examination and testing of this person's bowel will not reveal any abnormality. The symptom, nausea, is being generated at the level of the limbic system in the mind. It is just as real as a symptom caused by a problem in the stomach or small bowel, but it doesn't originate there. By interfering with the sensory input at the level of the brain, depression or anxiety can produce virtually any symptom.

5.1.3 Short circuit for physical symptoms

The short circuit analogy can be used here to help the patient understand. The limbic system is a key common pathway for sensory nerves to the cortex. The limbic system also plays a part in affecting the motor output nerves. The following diagram is an oversimplification but it does achieve one key purpose, which is to link mental illness to real physical symptoms.

Consider sharing this 'circuit diagram' with your patient.

Here the autonomic part of the peripheral nervous system is mostly affected. Whilst in a condition such as IBS there is no (currently) measurable pathology found in the end organ – in this case the gut – the circuitry can be affected 'upstream' creating abnormalities in the processing of nerve transmission, and generating symptoms. With the sympathetic and parasympathetic nervous system innervated, a series of physical symptoms can ensue – such as bloating, muscle spasms, changes to bowel habit and stool consistency.

Without this clearly described link, patients can find it confusing that their doctor is suggesting treatments linked with anxiety or depression for bowel symptoms. This can lead to poor compliance, disengagement with treatments and multiple visits for second opinions. It is not uncommon for patients to feel offended at the suggestion that mental health may have a link to their physical health symptoms.

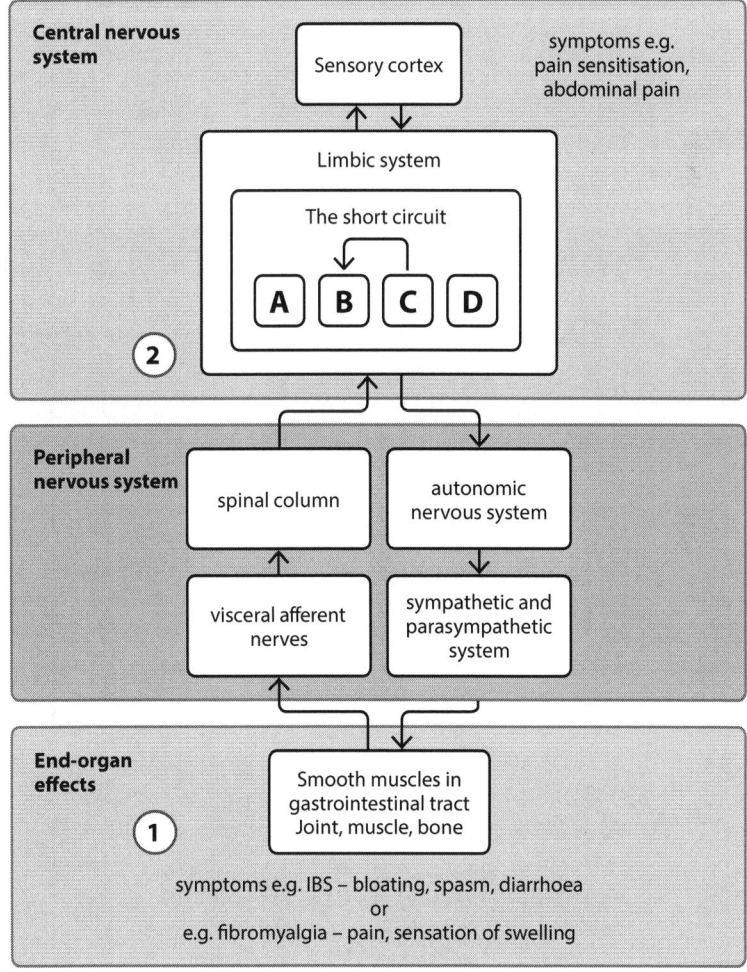

The symptoms felt and described by patients with say, fibromyalgia, are as real as those with osteoarthritis or rheumatoid arthritis. However, the position of the pathology is more likely to be 'higher' up the nerve pathway than other forms of arthritis.

Equally, with a condition like IBS, the bowel symptoms are significant but the contribution to this pathology may be influenced at the limbic system.

With this simple diagram, you can show the patient two clear and distinct treatment targets. At target 1, you are treating the 'downstream symptoms' and these will depend on the condition you are treating. At target 2, you are treating the mental health symptoms with treatment like SSRIs or CBT – but these will likely have an improvement on the physical symptoms of conditions like fibromyalgia or IBS.

5.2 Fibromyalgia

What you'll learn in this section
This section describes the classification, epidemiology, diagnosis and treatment of fibromyalgia as a disorder.

How this helps:
Fibromyalgia is a commonly seen illness which is often associated with a condition such as depression or anxiety. By helping your patient understand the connection, it will help them rationalise their illness and better engage with management.

The term fibromyalgia has only recently come into being. It was first used in the late 1970s and early 1980s. Over the years there has been considerable controversy as to its place in medical science. It has been described variously as a neurological, rheumatological, biochemical and psychosomatic condition. Some clinicians have even refused to acknowledge its existence as a disorder due to the fact that no chemical or radiographic abnormalities can be detected in such patients. For these reasons many patients can find it difficult to acknowledge the label and understand its origin and treatment for them personally.

When diagnosing fibromyalgia or treating a patient with the same it is therefore essential that you are able to convey the logical link between any symptom they have and the mental health associations.

Fibromyalgia is now generally understood as a medical condition characterised by chronic widespread pain and a heightened pain response to pressure. Other symptoms include tiredness, sleep problems, numbness and tingling, sensitivity to noise, lights or temperature, memory difficulties and muscle stiffness. It has also been associated with restless legs syndrome, irritable bowel syndrome and irritable bladder syndrome.

> Fibromyalgia can be described as the volume setting of the neurones being set too high, effectively increasing the 'noise' level of the neurones, resulting in the patient experiencing pain.

Fibromyalgia is strongly associated with depression, anxiety and post-traumatic stress disorder, amongst other common mental health disorders.

The assessment, diagnosis and treatment of a patient with fibromyalgia are grossly incomplete without thorough attention paid to the patient's mental health.

5.2.1 Epidemiology

Fibromyalgia affects between 2% and 8% of the population. Females are affected about twice as often as males. There is a higher rate if a first-degree relative also has the condition. It is also more commonly diagnosed in patients with chronic forms of arthritis, although it is unclear whether this has a causal association.

Some estimates suggest fibromyalgia may be undiagnosed in up to 75% of affected people.

5.2.2 Cause

The cause of fibromyalgia is unknown.

Sensitisation hypothesis

The evidence suggests that the pain in fibromyalgia results primarily from pain-processing pathways functioning abnormally. Sensitisation has been suggested as a possible mechanism.

People with fibromyalgia may have a lower threshold for pain due to errors in signal processing in the dorsal column of the spinal cord, the thalamus or the limbic system. Therefore a heightened sensation of pain is generated in the sensory cortex of the brain despite there not being the initial physical noxious stimulus at the site of the pain.

Neuropathic pain, major depressive disorder and anxiety often occur with fibromyalgia. Therefore it has been proposed that monoaminergic neurotransmitters may be involved. Others have proposed a role in the inflammatory cascade in producing symptoms. In vulnerable individuals, psychological stress or illness can cause abnormalities in inflammatory and stress pathways that regulate mood and pain.

In simple terms, ones that a patient can understand and relate to, it can be described as the volume setting of the neurones being set too high, effectively increasing the 'noise' level of the neurones, resulting in the patient experiencing pain. The fact that drugs such as SSRIs have a positive effect on fibromyalgia lends further evidence to this hypothesis.

5.2.3 Diagnosis

There is no single pathognomonic feature of fibromyalgia. There is no laboratory finding or biomarker that can diagnose fibromyalgia. There aren't even any clearly defined and approved diagnostic criteria.

American College of Rheumatology (ACR) criteria

The ACR originally used the 'tender points' test. This highlighted eighteen points on the patient's body, arranged in nine symmetrical pairs over the neck, clavicle, scapula, buttocks and limbs. The criteria included a minimum 'count' of tender points on the body.

However, these criteria have been completely dropped owing to their very poor specificity.

The 2010 revision includes, instead, the use of the widespread pain index (WPI) which counts up to nineteen general body areas in which the person has experienced pain in the preceding 2 weeks. It also uses the symptom severity (SS) scale. The SS scale rates the severity of the person's fatigue, unrefreshed waking, cognitive symptoms, and general somatic symptoms, each on a scale from 0 to 3, for a composite score ranging from 0–12. The ACR diagnostic criteria then include:

- WPI ≥7 and SS ≥5 OR WPI 3–6 and SS ≥9
- Symptoms have been present at a similar level for at least 3 months
- No other diagnosable disorder otherwise explains the pain.

This tends to be the most commonly used research tool but in clinical practice in the UK is rarely used in general practice. Most diagnosis relies on a systematic exclusion of other differentials and often practitioners will test for inflammatory markers and autoimmune biochemistry as excluders of inflammatory arthritis.

5.2.4 Differential diagnosis

It is useful to rule out the following before reaching a diagnosis of fibromyalgia:

- Arthritis
  - polymyalgia rheumatica
  - rheumatoid arthritis
  - ankylosing spondylitis
- Peripheral neuropathies
  - nerve compression
  - carpal tunnel syndrome
- Systemic disorders and vasculitis
  - systemic lupus erythematosus
  - Sjögren syndrome
  - hypothyroidism

- Neurological
  - multiple sclerosis
  - myasthenia gravis.

Fibromyalgia is not usually associated with synovial joint swelling (although patients may have a sensation of swelling) or a focal or dermatomal distribution of pain or sensory loss.

5.2.5 Treatment

Before considering any treatment for fibromyalgia it is vitally important that you fully explain to the patient what you understand the condition to be. The treatments may involve pain relief or other medication to deal with the symptoms; however, you will also need to address the underlying mental health condition. Without the patient fully understanding the link between the two, this suggestion of treatments normally associated with depression or anxiety can seem confusing and counterproductive to the patient. Using the circuit diagram in *Section 5.1* can be very helpful.

Painkillers

Painkillers are treating the final downstream symptom of fibromyalgia – pain. It is difficult, as a doctor, to deny a patient pain relief in a form that gives them the immediate relief they want and need. However, this is doing very little to address the 'upstream' causes of the syndrome, including any mental health disorder that may be present.

Whilst simple pain relief may have a role to play in the day-to-day improvement in a patient's ability to function, it is wholly inappropriate to simply continue up the pain treatment ladder – particularly the opioid ladder – without fully exploring options which have an impact on mental health. Many patients who end up being treated with higher-dose and more potent opioids reach a stage of tolerance and dependency and will often not achieve remission of the pain symptoms.

Most national medical associations and bodies recommend against the use of strong opioids but acknowledge there may be a place for weaker opioids as a short-term relief measure. Tramadol has been tested in many patients and found to be more effective than other opioids, leading some to suggest its specific benefits may be related to its serotonin action rather than its opioid action.

Exercise

There is strong evidence indicating that exercise improves fitness and sleep and may reduce pain and fatigue in some people with fibromyalgia. Cardiovascular exercise is effective for some people, and resistance training may improve pain in women.

Aerobic exercise for adults can be associated with an improved quality of life; it decreases pain and improves physical function whilst not worsening fatigue and stiffness.

The common recommendation is a graduated approach to an exercise programme, beginning with small, frequent exercise periods, and building up from there. Since exercise is associated with a range of other health benefits, all patients who are physically able to exercise should be encouraged to do so. If the pain of fibromyalgia is preventing the exercise, you should explain that by using a graduated approach, the patient will be able to overcome this and as the fibromyalgia pain subsides, so the exercise can become more intensive.

Cognitive behavioural therapy

In a 2020 Cochrane review[1] cognitive behavioural therapy was found to have a small but beneficial effect for reducing pain and distress. CBT has a well-evidenced beneficial effect on anxiety and depression and can be assumed, therefore, to improve symptoms of any 'downstream' effect on depression and anxiety such as fibromyalgia.

Effect sizes tend to be small when CBT is used as a stand-alone treatment for fibromyalgia patients, but these improve significantly when CBT is part of a wider treatment programme which includes pharmacology and graded exercise.

---

[1] Williams, A.C. de C., Fisher, E., Hearn, L. and Eccleston, C. (2020) Psychological therapies for the management of chronic pain (excluding headache) in adults. *Cochrane Database Systematic Rev.*, **8(8):** CD007407.

A 2010 systematic review[2] of CBT suggests it can also improve a patient's self-efficacy for coping with pain and reduces the number of doctor visits.

See *Section 6.4* for a detailed consideration of CBT.

Antidepressants

Antidepressants are associated with improvements in pain, depression, fatigue, sleep disturbances, and health-related quality of life in patients with fibromyalgia. The most commonly used antidepressants are SSRIs, followed closely by SNRIs. SSRIs are generally considered the first-line antidepressant therapy, including if the primary indicator for treatment is a secondary condition like fibromyalgia.

SNRIs such as duloxetine have also been associated with improvements in neuropathic pain and, as such, might be more suitable for patients with a primary mental health condition with an associated pain condition like fibromyalgia. Tricyclic antidepressants (TCAs), such as amitriptyline or nortriptyline, may also produce a dual effect like this. However, many people experience more adverse effects with TCAs and this will always need to be balanced with any possible benefit. It should also be noted that the treatment dose of TCAs for depression is significantly higher than the dose used for other conditions.

Patients should be counselled that the normal time to onset of benefit for SSRIs for depression and anxiety is 2–4 weeks; however, benefits in terms of the pain and stiffness associated with fibromyalgia can take up to 3 months before becoming apparent.

Anticonvulsant medication

The anticonvulsant medications gabapentin and pregabalin may be used to reduce pain and they can have a beneficial effect on anxiety. The effects of these drugs can vary significantly between patients and a therapeutic trial may be recommended to test the

[2] Bernardy, K., Füber, N., Köllner, V. and Häuser, W. (2010) Efficacy of cognitive-behavioral therapies in fibromyalgia syndrome – a systematic review and metaanalysis of randomized controlled trials. *J Rheumatol*, **37(10):** 1991–2005.

effectiveness. Side-effects can be troublesome in some patients, with gabapentin usually being more associated with adverse effects than pregabalin.

See *Section 6.5* for a detailed consideration of pharmacological therapies.

5.2.6 Course and prognosis

Fibromyalgia is a chronic relapsing condition. Some studies report that patients with fibromyalgia will consult, on average, ten times per year. The chronic pain and fatigue can contribute to obesity and associated medical risk factors.

A complete 'cure' is rare and most patients will go through a remitting/relapsing cycle, strongly associated with life stressors and mental health status.

The following factors usually indicate a poorer prognosis:

- Long-standing fibromyalgia
- Major psychiatric disease or severe depression and anxiety that responds poorly to treatment
- An ingrained pattern of work avoidance
- Marked functional impairment despite multidisciplinary approaches to treatment
- Opioid or alcohol dependence.

Fibromyalgia can be associated with morbidity and shortened life expectancy through a number of illnesses such as metabolic syndrome and diabetes. Suicide rates are higher amongst patients with depression and fibromyalgia.

5.3 Irritable bowel syndrome

What you'll learn in this section
This section describes the classification, epidemiology, diagnosis and treatment of IBS as a disorder.

> **How this helps**
> IBS is a commonly seen illness which is often associated with a condition such as depression or anxiety. By helping your patient understand the connection, it will help them rationalise their illness and better engage with management.

Irritable bowel syndrome (IBS) is a common disorder that affects the intestine. Its symptoms include cramping, abdominal pain, bloating, and diarrhoea or constipation, or both. IBS is often a long-term condition and can start in the early teens and last a lifetime. Symptoms can range from very mild to very severe and for most sufferers this illness can significantly affect quality of life.

IBS is strongly associated with depression, anxiety and other common mental health disorders. It is not known whether these have a direct causal effect on each other but the association is clear. It is also known that the treatment for the anxiety or depression can significantly improve bowel symptoms. The assessment and management of a patient with IBS is therefore incomplete without due care and attention to the mental health status.

IBS is considered a functional disorder in that it causes chronic abdominal complaints without a structural or biochemical cause that could explain symptoms.

5.3.1 Epidemiology

In most populations, women report more IBS symptoms than men, with rates in women 1.5- to 3-fold higher than those seen in men. However, in South Asia, South America and Africa, rates of IBS in men are much closer to those of women, and in some cases higher.

IBS occurs in all age groups, including children and the elderly. 50% of patients with IBS report having first had symptoms before the age of 35 years. Patients aged over 50 years report milder pain, but their overall quality of life is worse.

IBS can be associated with lower socioeconomic status, a finding supported by the theory that lower income is associated with poorer healthcare outcomes, lower overall quality of life, and increased life stressors. However, some studies have suggested that the opposite is true. Being in a higher socioeconomic group during childhood could be associated with higher prevalence of IBS. In some studies, people in professional and managerial roles were found to have higher overall rates of IBS[3].

The relative risk of IBS is twice as high in individuals with a biological relative with IBS. Having a mother or father with IBS is an independent risk factor for an individual having IBS and a stronger predictor than having a twin with IBS.

5.3.2 Cause

The cause of IBS remains unknown; however, it is postulated to arise from abnormalities in the gut–brain interaction and the visceral nervous system.

Stress, anxiety and depression

Depression or anxiety precede IBS symptoms in about two-thirds of people with IBS. These mental health conditions can predispose previously healthy people to developing IBS after a bout of gastroenteritis.

The assessment and management of a patient with IBS is incomplete without due care and attention to their mental health status.

Psychological factors, such as depression or anxiety, have not been shown to conclusively cause or influence the onset of IBS, but definitely play a role in the persistence, severity of symptoms and impact on quality of life. Childhood physical and psychological abuse is associated with the development of IBS.

It is proposed that an abnormality of the stress response, involving the hypothalamic–pituitary–adrenal axis (HPA) and the sympathetic nervous system, is responsible for IBS symptoms. Both of these have been shown to be abnormal in people with IBS.

---

[3] Canavan, C., West, J. and Card, T. (2014) The epidemiology of irritable bowel syndrome. *Clin Epidemiol*, **6**: 71–80.

Post-infection and bacterial overgrowth

Approximately 10% of IBS cases are triggered by an acute gastro-enteritis infection. Increased gut permeability is associated with IBS and it is postulated that the release of high levels of proinflammatory cytokines during acute infection causes increased gut permeability, leading to bacteria crossing the epithelial barrier. This then results in damage to local tissues and an autoimmune response.

Small intestinal bacterial overgrowth (SIBO) occurs with greater frequency in people who have been diagnosed with IBS compared to healthy controls, and relative abundance of commensal bacteria has been implied but by no means proven. The association with fungal and protozoan microbes has also been studied, without a definite causal association being found.

Food intolerance

True food allergy is rare and is a different pathology to IBS. The link between food products and IBS is complex and unclear. It has been suggested that lack of fibre is the cause; however, this is not well-evidenced. The addition of soluble fibre to the diet may improve some symptoms of irritable bowel, but no strong association exists for sufferers of IBS and generally low dietary fibre intake. Some patients will find that certain foods can trigger episodes of IBS but they may find it difficult to generate a definitive pattern, and the pattern does not seem to hold true across different patients generally. For this reason it is difficult to implicate food and diet specifically as a cause for IBS.

5.3.3 Diagnosis

No specific laboratory or imaging tests can diagnose irritable bowel syndrome. Diagnosis should be based on symptoms and the exclusion of other pathology.

Features more associated with other organic pathology:

- Onset at >50 years of age
- Weight loss
- Blood in the stool

- Iron-deficiency anaemia
- Nocturnal symptoms
- Family history of colon cancer, coeliac disease or inflammatory bowel disease.

It is usual to perform blood tests for inflammatory markers, thyroid hormone, immune markers (e.g. coeliac disease) and iron profiles. Abnormalities in these are not associated with IBS. Faecal calprotectin tests can help distinguish inflammatory bowel disease from irritable bowel syndrome.

Rome criteria

The Rome IV criteria include recurrent abdominal pain, on average, at least one day per week in the last 3 months, associated with two or more of the following further criteria:

- Pain related to defecation
- Associated with a change in frequency of stool
- Associated with a change in form (appearance) of stool.

The symptom onset should be at least 6 months before diagnosis.

5.3.4 Differential diagnosis

Before making a diagnosis, the clinician should feel satisfied that the following are excluded or highly unlikely, given the set of symptoms (not an exhaustive list):

- Colon cancer
- Inflammatory bowel disease
- Thyroid disorders (hyper- or hypothyroidism)
- Giardiasis
- Coeliac disease
- Less commonly:
  - carcinoid syndrome
  - microscopic colitis
  - bacterial overgrowth
  - eosinophilic gastroenteritis.

5.3.5 Treatment

Referencing the short circuit diagram in *Section 5.1*, there are two potential treatment targets – those that act at the bowel and those that act on the mental health element.

Dietary

Low FODMAP diet

FODMAPs are fermentable oligo-, di-, monosaccharides and polyols. These are poorly absorbed in the small intestine and subsequently fermented by the bacteria in the distal small and proximal large intestine. A 2018 systematic review[4] found that although there is evidence of improved IBS symptoms with a low FODMAP diet, the evidence is of very low quality. The restriction of FODMAPs necessarily means the restriction of gluten, so positive results may be as a result of undiagnosed coeliac disease.

Fibre

Some evidence suggests that soluble fibre supplementation (e.g. psyllium/ispaghula husk) is effective by acting as a bulking agent, and generates a more consistent stool. This can be helpful for patients with both diarrhoea- and constipation-predominant IBS.

However, insoluble fibre (e.g. bran) has not been found to be effective for IBS and in some cases may even aggravate symptoms. Overall the evidence for fibre is weak and although it may improve stool consistency and softness, it probably doesn't improve pain.

Target 1 - Gut

Antispasmodics

Antispasmodics can be divided into two groups – those acting as anticholinergics and those acting directly on the smooth muscle.

Anticholinergics include **dicycloverine** and **hyoscine**, which act on the parasympathetic system and can improve pain, bloating

---

[4] Dionne, J., Ford, A.C., Yuan, Y. *et al.* (2018) A systematic review and meta-analysis evaluating the efficacy of a gluten-free diet and a low FODMAPs diet in treating symptoms of irritable bowel syndrome. *Am J Gastroenterol*, **113(9)**: 1290–1300.

and diarrhoea symptoms. As anticholinergics they can display typical side-effects such as dry mouth, tachycardia and difficulty passing urine.

Mebeverine acts directly on the smooth muscle and has no anticholinergic activity. It therefore has the advantage of not producing anticholinergic side-effects.

Peppermint oil also appears to be useful as an antispasmodic. Studies have suggested that, in the short term, it is significantly superior to placebo in improving a number of IBS symptoms.

Target 2 – Mental health

Cognitive behavioural therapy

Psychological therapies as a whole have demonstrated good efficacy in reducing the severity of IBS symptoms. CBT has been tested most rigorously in multiple RCTs and demonstrates significant and durable effects on IBS symptoms and quality of life.

NICE[5] recommends that referral for psychological interventions should be considered for people with IBS who do not respond to pharmacological treatments after 12 months and who develop a pattern of chronic relapsing symptoms. Other psychological interventions such as hypnosis are considered to be acceptable by NICE, although evidence in this area is poor and services generally not available on the NHS.

CBT works through exposure management and training the patient through behavioural adaption to relieve the emotional impact of the illness.

For a more detailed review of CBT see *Section 6.4.*

Low-dose tricyclics

TCAs have a better evidence base than SSRIs for IBS treatment. The low doses recommended by NICE are considered as second-line treatment for people with IBS if laxatives, loperamide or antispasmodics have not helped.

---

[5] NICE (2008, updated 2017) *Irritable bowel syndrome in adults: diagnosis and management.* Clinical guideline [CG61].

NICE suggests 5–10mg equivalent of amitriptyline, taken once at night, with the dose not usually increasing beyond 30mg. At this dose, the TCA is unlikely to be having any direct antidepression effect but these drugs have been shown to have an impact on functional IBS symptoms such as pain and bloating.

SSRIs

The evidence base for SSRI usage is not strong and NICE recommends further research in this area. However, the American College of Gastroenterology[6], after an extensive research review, concluded that there is enough research support on the effectiveness of both TCAs and SSRIs.

SSRIs have been found to have a positive effect on gut motility and visceral hypersensitivity, although further research is ongoing.

SSRIs remain the first-line pharmacological treatment for any patient with a separate diagnosis of depression or anxiety. It is not entirely clear yet whether the improvement in IBS symptoms is a direct effect of the drugs or whether the IBS symptoms improve because of an improvement in anxiety or depression as a secondary effect.

See *Section 6.5* for a detailed consideration of pharmacological therapies.

5.3.6 Course and prognosis

Irritable bowel syndrome tends to be a lifelong chronic condition with a relapsing and remitting course. The illness will often follow the course of the patient's mental health status. Some patients may have long symptom-free periods interspersed with periods of severe symptoms. When this does happen, it is important to be vigilant for a new underlying diagnosis. Irritable bowel syndrome is not associated directly with mortality and does not shorten lifespan.

---

[6] Lacy, B.E., Pimentel, M., Brenner, D. *et al.* (2021) ACG Clinical Guideline: management of irritable bowel syndrome. *American Journal of Gastroenterology*, **116(1):** 17–44.

5.4 Chronic pain syndrome

What you'll learn in this section

This section describes the classification, epidemiology, diagnosis and treatment of chronic pain syndrome as a disorder.

How this helps

Chronic pain syndrome is a commonly-seen illness which is often associated with a condition such as depression or anxiety. By helping your patient understand the connection, it will help them rationalise their illness and better engage with management.

Chronic pain syndrome (CPS) is a common problem that is poorly defined and understood. Generally speaking, the accepted definition is of pain that has lasted longer than 12 months or pain that persists longer than the reasonably expected healing time.

CPS is a constellation of syndromes that usually do not respond well to the typical pain and analgesia ladder. The condition is strongly associated with mental health conditions such as depression and anxiety and its treatment is incomplete without a thorough consideration of the mental health effects.

The underlying origin of the pain can be from any organ system of the body but is most commonly musculoskeletal or rheumatological. Neurological, urological and gastroenterological organs are also often affected. It is outside the scope of this book to address the physical aspects of these individually. Nevertheless, they can all result in a chronic pain syndrome with certain similar features.

5.4.1 Epidemiology

In the UK, chronic pain affects anywhere from 8% to 15% of the population. It affects women at a higher rate than men, and is responsible for about 4.6 million primary consultations each year[7].

In the USA, chronic pain has been estimated to occur in approximately 30% of the population; 34% for women and 26% for men.

5.4.2 Cause

The primary origin of the pain usually comes from a pathologically affected organ. However, some patients respond well to traditional strategies whilst others develop CPS.

The pathophysiology of chronic pain syndrome is multifactorial and complex and is still poorly understood. Patients with concurrent mental illness such as major depression or anxiety are prone to developing CPS. Various neuromuscular, reproductive, gastrointestinal (GI) and urologic disorders may cause or contribute to chronic pain. Sometimes multiple organic contributing factors may be present in a single patient.

Pain sensitisation

It is postulated that a persistent activation of pain signals to the dorsal horn may produce a pain sensitisation effect. This lowers the threshold for pain signals to be transmitted. Nerve fibres (particularly C fibres that have a slow conductivity) may even begin to generate and transmit pain signals. In chronic pain, this process is difficult to reverse or stop once established.

Chronic pain syndrome likely involves brain structure and function as well as nerve function. Persistent pain has been shown to cause grey matter loss, which is reversible once the pain has resolved – likely explained by neuroplasticity.

Dysfunction of neurotransmitters such as dopamine and serotonin – which have been implicated in both depression and altered pain sensation – could potentially act as a shared mechanism between chronic pain and mental health disorders.

---

[7] Belsey, J. (2002) Primary care workload in the management of chronic pain: a retrospective cohort study using a GP database to identify resource implications for UK primary care. *Journal of Medical Economics*, **5**: 39–50.

Risk factors

The following factors are associated with a higher risk, although they are by no means exclusive or exhaustive:

- Increased deprivation
- Increased age
- Female sex
- Lower educational attainment
- Higher BMI
- Poorer mental health status
- Sedentary lifestyle.

5.4.3 Diagnosis

There is no universally accepted definition of chronic pain and many classifications exist, none of which has found universal favour. Chronic pain has been classified by some as pain that lasts longer than 3–6 months. Other researchers have placed the transition from acute to chronic pain at 12 months. An alternative definition of chronic pain, involving no fixed duration, is "pain that extends beyond the expected period of healing".

Chronic pain syndrome occurs in up to 25% of patients with chronic pain. Chronic pain syndrome includes both the physical effects of the pain and also a mental health element such as anxiety or depression.

The diagnosis is usually a clinical one, as no formal diagnostic criteria exist.

5.4.4 Management

It is often the case that by treating the physical pain with pain-relieving medicines without appropriate treatment of the mental health element, neither the physical pain nor the mental side will improve.

I often use this analogy to help patients understand the connection between physical pain and mental illness:

> ### Consultation tip – the guitar and the amp
>
> Ask your patient to think of the sound from an electric guitar as representing the original source of pain. Then tell your patient that the pain is related to the loudness of the sound – the louder the sound, the more pain they feel. The guitar alone makes some sound, but it is made significantly louder when played through an amplifier. A mental health disorder acts like an amplifier – it doesn't cause the pain in the first place but it does affect the amount of pain felt. Suffering with a coexisting disorder like anxiety or depression turns the volume on the amp right up. By treating the mental illness, you turn down the amplifier, therefore reducing the perception of pain.

This is likely to be true in the reverse case – if you address only the mental health side without appropriate analgesia, there may not be an improvement in either.

Once both mental health and pain are addressed, through appropriate management, patients will often see an improvement in both.

It is outside the scope of this book to discuss analgesic pain relief measures in any detail. These will, of course, vary hugely with the nature of the underlying condition. Patients may well be under the care of a medical or surgical specialist such as a rheumatologist or neurologist.

A note on opioids

Opioids can, and do, provide some pain relief. However, a recently published NICE guideline[8] on chronic pain management has suggested that GPs do not use opioids as an option, even in the short term, for chronic pain.

The NICE committee points to the lack of evidence (albeit with caveats and limitations) for effectiveness of opioids, along with evidence of long-term harm, to recommend against opioid use.

Long-term use of high doses of opioids has been linked with depression.

---

[8] NICE (2021) *Chronic pain (primary and secondary) in over 16s: assessment of all chronic pain and management of chronic primary pain* [NG193].

Patients who are already on opioids in the long term from a chronic pain syndrome can be started on a regime to lower the dose and eventually remove them; however, it should be noted that this may take some time. The tapering to a more appropriate pharmacological agent, such as an SSRI, will increase the chances of a successful taper and stopping of the opioid.

In terms of the mental health side there are a number of interventions with an evidence base.

Physical therapy

Exercise and physical therapy has some evidence base for the reduction of chronic pain and should be suggested and encouraged. If a locally commissioned group exercise programme is available then this should be offered.

Clearly there are numerous other long-term health benefits to exercise, making this a very easy option to encourage – if, of course, your patient is physically able to do it. Exercise is shown to improve mood as well as chronic pain scores.

Cognitive behavioural therapy

See *Section 6.4* for a detailed consideration of CBT.

CBT has been shown in some cases to improve pain scores. It is not certain whether this is a direct effect on the pain or an indirect effect though improvement of the mental health effects of the chronic pain syndrome.

Acceptance and commitment therapy

The 2021 NICE guidance for chronic pain also recommends acceptance and commitment therapy (ACT) as a possible psychological intervention for chronic pain patients. ACT is a form of psychotherapy based on psychological intervention that uses acceptance and mindfulness strategies. It includes commitment and behaviour-change strategies, to increase psychological flexibility.

ACT uses a concept of workability – simply put, finding out what works for the patient, in order to take a step towards the values and feelings that matter to them. Its therapeutic effect is a positive spiral where feeling better leads to a better understanding of what works.

Acupuncture

The same NICE guidance recommends acupuncture as a possible intervention. It points to 27 studies which have shown short-term benefits in reduction of pain and improved quality of life. These benefits are shown to last up to 3 months; however, evidence for any longer-term improvement is lacking.

Acupuncture is not universally (or even widely) available on the NHS but many specialist pain management clinics and some physiotherapy departments do have access to it.

Interventions not recommended by NICE

The following were not recommended, or had a recommendation for further research due to lack of evidence:

- TENS therapy
- Ultrasound
- Interferential therapy
- Manual therapy
- Hypnosis.

Pharmacological treatments

NICE has reported that the evidence indicates that antidepressants across the classes of SSRIs, SNRIs and TCAs (e.g. duloxetine, amitriptyline, fluoxetine, paroxetine, citalopram and sertraline) improve quality of life, pain and psychological distress compared with placebo. Most of these trials have been specifically for fibromyalgia but NICE was satisfied that the results could be generalised for chronic pain syndromes.

Duloxetine had a larger amount of long-term evidence of effectiveness. However, there is very little in the way of head-to-head comparisons and as such, there is no particular preference for which antidepressant to use.

It should be noted that SSRIs and SNRIs are not licensed for chronic pain. However, since chronic pain syndromes will have an element of a mental health condition (for which they are licensed), they can often be used within their licence.

See *Section 6.5* for a detailed consideration of pharmacological therapies.

5.4.5 Course and prognosis

Chronic pain syndrome is, as its name implies, a long-term condition that has a strong propensity to worsen without intervention.

Given that there is no medical intervention, pharmacological or non-pharmacological, that is helpful for more than a minority of people with chronic pain, and benefits of treatments are modest in terms of effect size and duration, the condition provides a major challenge for healthcare providers.

5.5 Chronic fatigue syndrome

What you'll learn in this section
This section describes the classification, epidemiology, diagnosis and treatment of CFS as a disorder.

How this helps
CFS is a commonly-seen complex, chronic medical illness. It can be associated with a number of comorbid conditions such as depression and anxiety, the treatment of which may help your patient cope with the symptoms of CFS.

Chronic fatigue syndrome (CFS), also called myalgic encephalomyelitis (ME), is a complex, long-term medical condition involving a broad range of symptoms. Diagnosis is based on a syndromic set of the patient's symptoms – no confirmatory diagnostic test is available.

Since this is the case, it is a subject of much debate and differing opinion amongst physicians, researchers and patient advocates. Each group can often promote a different name, diagnostic criteria, causative agent and treatment. Evidence of proposed causes and treatments remains poor, contradictory or non-existent.

The condition is primarily characterised by an overwhelming fatigue which is not due to ongoing exertion, is not relieved by rest, and is not attributable to another medical condition. Whilst fatigue is a common symptom in many illnesses, the unexplained fatigue and severity of functional impairment distinguishes CFS from those other illnesses.

CFS, whilst being a separate entity, is associated with the coexistence of mental health disorders such as depression and anxiety.

CFS, whilst being a separate entity, is associated with the coexistence of mental health disorders such as depression and anxiety, hence its appearance in this book. It is yet to be fully established whether one has a direct causative effect on the other – nevertheless, many mental health therapies can be effective for day-to-day management of CFS symptoms, even though they are by no means curative.

The assessment of a patient with CFS should always include enquiry as to their mental health status.

5.5.1 Epidemiology

Whilst studies vary in their diagnostic criteria, it is believed that about 1% of primary care patients have CFS. Around 250 000 people in the United Kingdom have CFS. Some studies quote a much higher figure, largely due to the differing diagnostic criteria used in the various studies. It is 1.5–2 times more common in women than in men.

It most commonly affects adults between the ages of 40 and 60 years; however, it can occur at any age, including in childhood. Chronic fatigue syndrome can be a major cause of school absence in older adolescents.

5.5.2 Cause

The cause of CFS is unknown. Several genetic, physiological and psychological factors are thought to work together to precipitate the condition. There are no biological markers for CFS, although this does not rule out the possibility that they exist.

There is a propensity for some cases to be preceded by a viral illness such as influenza or infectious mononucleosis, leading some to suggest that an infective or inflammatory cause may exist.

Risk factors

- Caucasians are diagnosed more frequently (although there may be confounding reasons for this)
- Female sex
- Age between 40 and 60
- First-degree relative with CFS
- Psychological stress and childhood trauma
- Perfectionist personalities
- Low physical fitness
- Pre-existing depressive and anxiety disorders.

5.5.3 Diagnosis

In October 2021 NICE published an update to the ME/CFS guidance[9]. The release of the new guidelines had been delayed to allow for further stakeholder meetings. The previous guidelines date back to 2007 and the newly-published guidance offers some significant changes – particularly relating to treatment modalities.

There is no test to diagnose CFS. The diagnosis is based on a syndromic set of symptoms and exclusion of more likely causes.

A diagnosis of CFS is made when symptoms cannot be explained by another cause and have lasted for:

- 3 months persistently in an adult
- 3 months in a child or young person (the diagnosis should be made in consultation with a paediatrician).

The key symptoms are:

---

[9] NICE (2021) *Myalgic encephalomyelitis (or encephalopathy)/chronic fatigue syndrome: diagnosis and management.* NICE guideline [NG206].

- Debilitating fatigue that is worsened by activity, is not caused by excessive cognitive, physical, emotional or social exertion, and is not significantly relieved by rest
- Post-exertional malaise after activity in which the worsening of symptoms:
  - is often delayed in onset by hours or days
  - is disproportionate to the activity
  - has a prolonged recovery time that may last hours, days, weeks or longer
- Unrefreshing sleep or sleep disturbance (or both), which may include:
  - feeling exhausted, feeling flu-like and stiff on waking
  - broken or shallow sleep, altered sleep pattern or hyper-somnia
- Cognitive difficulties (sometimes described as 'brain fog'), which may include problems finding words or numbers, difficulty in speaking, slowed responsiveness, short-term memory problems, and difficulty concentrating or multitasking.

- Other symptoms that can be present but are not exclusive to CFS/ME:

- Orthostatic intolerance and autonomic dysfunction, including dizziness, palpitations, fainting, nausea on standing or sitting upright from a reclining position
- Temperature hypersensitivity resulting in profuse sweating, chills, hot flushes, or feeling very cold
- Neuromuscular symptoms, including twitching and myo-clonic jerks
- Flu-like symptoms, including sore throat, tender glands, nausea, chills or muscle aches
- Intolerance to alcohol, or to certain foods and chemicals
- Heightened sensory sensitivities, including to light, sound, touch, taste and smell
- Pain, including pain on touch, myalgia, headaches, eye pain, abdominal pain or joint pain without acute redness, swelling or effusion.

If a child or young person under 18 years old has symptoms of possible CFS/ME they should be referred to a paediatrician. In many areas, a specialist ME/CFS team will be available for referral to, which will normally be staffed by a full multidisciplinary team including some or all of: physicians, physiotherapists, exercise physiologists, occupational therapists, dietitians, and clinical or counselling psychologists.

Differential diagnosis

Fatigue can be a very general and non-specific feature of many diseases and as such, the presentation of a patient with fatigue should also explore the possibility of:

- infectious diseases (e.g. Epstein–Barr virus, influenza, HIV infection)
- endocrine disorders (e.g. hypothyroidism)
- anaemia and haematological disease (e.g. lymphoma)
- rheumatological disease (e.g. polymyalgia rheumatica, rheumatoid arthritis)
- mental illnesses (e.g. depression)
- neurological diseases (e.g. multiple sclerosis)
- respiratory obstruction (e.g. obstructive sleep apnoea)
- others (such as autoimmune diseases, some chronic illness, alcohol or substance abuse, pharmacological side-effects, heavy metal exposure and toxicity, marked body weight fluctuation, nasal obstruction from allergies, sinusitis or anatomical obstruction).

Usual tests for exclusion of other diagnosis include:

- urinalysis for protein, blood and glucose
- full blood count, urea and electrolytes, liver function test, thyroid function test, erythrocyte sedimentation rate, C-reactive protein, HbA1c, screening blood tests for gluten sensitivity, serum calcium, serum ferritin levels (children and young people only)
- where indicated, rheumatoid factor, antinuclear antibodies, autoimmune tests
- some symptoms may require further tests, e.g. EMG, EEG, ECG, exclusion of inflammatory bowel disease.

5.5.4 Management

The treatment of CFS can be difficult and unrewarding.

The new NICE guidance is forthright in saying that there is no definitive proven treatment or cure for CFS.

Energy management

From 2007, NICE recommended graded exercise therapy (GET) and suggested that this should be delivered only by a suitably trained therapist with experience in CFS/ME. In most areas this would be provided under the wing of a physiotherapy service.

Under GET the patient undergoes planned increases in the duration of physical activity. The intensity should then be increased when appropriate, leading to aerobic exercise. This can take weeks, months or even years to achieve goals.

However, given a more recent review, the 2021 guidance no longer recommends this approach due to the significant number of cases of harm to patients from pushing outside of their exercise tolerance limits. Patients can be advised to assess their 'energy envelope' – the amount of physical exertion they can do without bringing on fatigue symptoms.

Graduated physical exercise programmes which fit the above definition are now not advised by NICE for most patients unless they are ready to progress their physical activity beyond their current activities of daily living.

Nevertheless, patients should be advised to exercise within their 'energy envelope' to the best of their ability. Given the potential harm from pushing this envelope, those patients who wish to progress in their physical energy management should be referred to an appropriate service. This can be done under the supervision of a CFS clinic with specialised physical therapists.

Cognitive behavioural therapy

See *Section 6.4* for a detailed consideration of CBT.

Previously NICE recommended that all patients with CFS receive CBT. However, more recent evidence is less favourable and now the advice is to only offer CBT to people with CFS who would like to use it to support them in managing their symptoms and to reduce the psychological distress associated with having a chronic illness.

It is important that you explain that CBT does not assume people have 'abnormal' illness beliefs and behaviours as an underlying cause of their CFS, but recognises that thoughts, feelings, behaviours and physiology interact with each other. You should explain that CBT is not curative of CFS but can help with the management of certain symptoms.

Pharmacology

Whilst SSRIs and low-dose TCAs have been trialled, the results are very inconclusive and inconsistent. The 2021 NICE guidance does not advise these medicines to treat CFS. However, it does suggest that any comorbid anxiety, depression or mood disorder be treated in the usual way.

5.5.5 Course and prognosis

Without any intervention, the full recovery rate is as low as 5%. In some studies return to work for those unable to work was between 8% and 30%.

Interestingly, a better outcome was associated with those patients who did not attribute illness to a different cause, and those having a sense of control over symptoms. Other indicators of better outcomes are younger age at diagnosis and lower fatigue severity at onset of the illness.

CFS can have a relapsing/remitting course and is often a lifelong illness. During a relapse (which can last from weeks to months) patients may be advised to lessen their physical activity and reassess their 'energy envelope'.

Chapter 6

Treating the patient

6.1 Management approaches

Treating the patient for a mental illness can only really begin in earnest once a diagnosis has been made and accepted by the patient. Of course, in this field, the diagnosis of illness is not simply a case of presence or absence of pathology. For example, no two patients with depression are the same. People differ in the type of symptoms they display, whether physical or psychological, the severity of the symptoms and the functional impact on their daily lives. Equally, no two patients live the same life. Lifestyle, social circumstances, work, family and other factors must all come into play when considering a treatment suitable for any one patient. In contrast with other medical illnesses, mental health treatment also comes with its own set of significant preconceptions and stigmas.

6.1.1 'That route'

'I don't want to go down that route' is a phrase we hear regularly in our day-to-day jobs in primary care. It could be in relation to getting a diagnosis of any form of mental illness; getting treatment – pills or therapy; it being documented on the medical notes; or even that they might start considering it as a contributing factor to their symptoms.

I sometimes get a little perplexed as to what 'that route' is. But a moment's consideration is probably all it needs to realise exactly what the patient is talking about. 'That route' seems to be an amalgamation of all the preconceptions and judgements about mental illness. Going down 'that route' involves being labelled as 'mad' or 'crazy', believing that their symptoms are 'all in the head' and that they are somehow to blame for their predicament.

Further down 'that route' would involve a stain on their records – if they were to seek help from another doctor, he or she might prejudge them as a 'time waster' or 'hypochondriac'. Furthermore, any attempt to find new employment would be made more difficult by the fact that the new employer would see them as unreliable or 'trouble'.

> In contrast with other medical illnesses, mental health treatment also comes with its own set of significant preconceptions and stigmas.

Wander further down the same path and you might be faced with actually being treated for a mental illness. At this point you might be taking pills or going through counselling or therapy. The pills are seemingly particularly damning. The commonly held belief would have the patient imagine themselves to be being 'propped up' by these chemicals. Reliance and addiction would soon follow and the long struggle to 'get off' them would be far more troublesome than any short-term gain they might produce. Also, the concept of any benefit is that it would be highly artificial and it certainly wouldn't address the underlying cause. They may even be dangerous in that they might mask another disease process, blinding both patient and doctor who walk together into disaster – missing another important diagnosis.

Therapy, depending on the patient's views, can seem even worse than the pills. This is seen as a touchy-feely technique to rid the patient of their 'issues'. It's useful for people who have had major trauma, physical or emotional, in their lives and if that doesn't apply to the patient then it would be a waste of time.

Well, considering all of the above, if it were true, I would certainly not want to go down 'that route' either. It's difficult to imagine that any right-thinking person would willingly set off at all!

It is important that you as the clinician hear, acknowledge, challenge and educate about these things being misinformation. Without this very important step right at the beginning of the patient's journey back to wellness, they are far less likely to achieve the results they want and need. Compliance with treatments will be far greater in those who have a good understanding of the treatments they are receiving. Patients feel more empowered when they know what's going on and much better able to recognise the success or failure of their treatment plans.

Imagine a world in which no one would want to go down 'that route' of treating asthma. Those with the condition would be so put off by the notion that they might have it, and so opposed to any form of treatment that the condition simply got worse and worse. It really wouldn't be long before they started to get very ill and it wouldn't be long before people started to die unnecessarily. Even if this extreme point wasn't reached there would undoubtedly be many people whose lives were so controlled by their asthma that they could not enjoy a fulfilled life. They might be limited in their ability to exercise and engage with sport and they might start subconsciously changing their life plans to fit in with what they could and couldn't do. This would be a shameful situation, as with the proper treatment, many asthmatics will live entirely normal lives and some asthmatics compete in the top-flight of many sporting disciplines.

Well, if it were true, I would certainly not want to go down 'that route' either. It's difficult to imagine that any right-thinking person would willingly set off at all!

The asthma consultation would also be fundamentally different. Many clinicians will recognise that a minority of patients, parents of children with asthma and family members of those with asthma, hold incorrect beliefs about inhalers. This might include the notion that the inhaler is addictive or somehow causes long-term damage to the lungs. If this was a majority-held belief then the clinician would have the extra job with almost every patient of unpicking and unravelling this. The consultation would take longer and compliance would naturally be much lower.

I believe that time spent at the beginning of the patient's journey with you as a clinician in exploring any concerns or beliefs around mental health or its treatment is time very well spent. It is likely to make further engagements more productive and hopefully help the patient be more involved in the decision-making regarding their own care. A quick hurried consultation when first diagnosing somebody with a mental illness or prescribing a drug for this is likely to be an extremely false economy, with a higher rate of relapse and re-consultation and a lower rate of compliance.

Case study - Jonah

Jonah is a 44-year-old mechanic who recently left service in the Royal Navy as an engineer. He and his wife have struggled to have children and after some failed cycles of IVF they are considering adoption. He presents to his GP, initially with poor sleep, excess tiredness during the day, bouts of anger and irritability and loss of libido.

Jonah's GP has examined him and performed blood tests to exclude a biochemical abnormality. The doctor, after performing a PHQ-9, suggests to Jonah that this could be a mental health issue – namely depression – and that she would like to explore it further.

Jonah: *'Are you suggesting antidepressants? I'm not keen on that thank you – I've seen plenty of people on antidepressants. I'm not that sort and I don't want to be addicted.'*

Doctor: *'If you are suffering from depression, there are lots of different types of treatment – many people can be treated entirely with talking therapies so you won't automatically be offered pills.*

If you are offered pills, it may surprise you to hear they are not addictive. Antidepressants are the sort of medicine that get talked about a lot and unfortunately a lot of stuff out there about them is simply not true.

I want to make sure you make the right choice for you. It's not really my place to tell you what to do, but it is my job to ensure you have all the right information about all the different options available, so that you can make an informed choice. You are much more likely to get a better outcome if you make your choice based on good quality, correct information and I can give that to you.'

Jonah: *'But I am going through assessments for adoption – it will look bad if I have a diagnosis of depression and I certainly don't want them to know I'm taking antidepressants.'*

Doctor: *'It's a common worry, but it's not something you need to worry about. Employers, agencies and council services will not discriminate on the basis of ill health – in fact many people with a mental illness can and do adopt.*

> *What they will want to see is that you are looking after your health, making sure you are seeing the doctor when you need to and getting the appropriate help.*
>
> *Getting treatment for depression won't be seen as a sign of weakness or inability to adopt; in fact social services would be more concerned if you are ill and are not engaging in sensible recommended treatments.'*

Jonah, having heard reassurances, is now in a much better place to listen to the different treatment options, their pros and cons and can go on to make a personal plan with his doctor.

Consultation tip

Try telling the David Beckham story. David Beckham is a very rich, famous and successful man. But many people don't know that he has suffered with asthma. Imagine if David Beckham had not gone down 'that route' of treating his asthma. Imagine if the treatment for asthma was frowned upon and stigmatised and those suffering from asthma were encouraged to just get on with it.

If this were the case, David Beckham would still have been an extremely talented athlete and footballer. However, he would not have reached the pinnacle of his sporting discipline. He wouldn't have turned professional at all and we certainly wouldn't know who he was.

In reality, David got some treatment for his asthma. The treatment didn't change him or give him something he didn't already have – it just took away the pathology. He went on to achieve fame in his sport.

The same could be said for a mental health condition. Why should people not attempt to treat the condition rather than live under its burden and fail to reach their true potential?

6.1.2 Treating the short circuit

As has been described, the short circuit tool is helpful in reducing stigma and helping the patient separate an illness from their sense of self. It is an explanatory tool to help mental health treatment become more accessible and less frightening for patients. Whilst the short circuit tool does not promote one method of therapy over another, it is definitely helpful to the patient with whom you have just used the short circuit tool to explain how and where the various treatments relate to the model.

The short circuit tool is just an elegant way to visualise an invisible illness. Once the pathology is visualised as the short circuit, you can point to a diagram and explain to the patient that their treatments will target this.

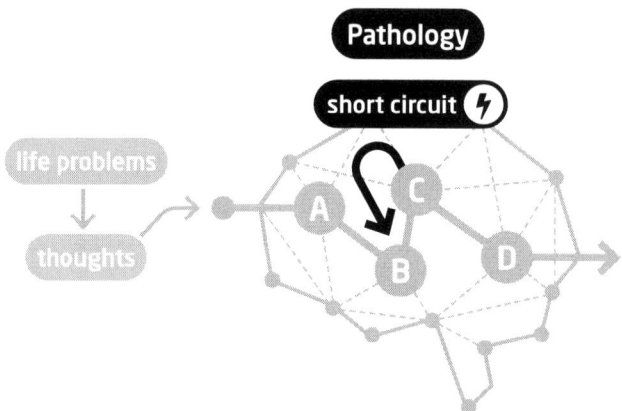

Using the short circuit model, in order to treat pathology, the short circuit must be broken. By doing this, irrespective of life pressures continuing, the symptoms of the mental illness will be relieved.

In the following sections, a number of different therapeutic interventions will be described. Relating these back to the short circuit tool, they can be categorised into those that 'break' the short circuit and therefore can be considered treatments for the underlying mental illness, and those that work further 'downstream' and work by relieving some symptom of the mental illness.

This list is not exhaustive but it can be useful in explaining to the patient where a medicine or therapeutic intervention works by pointing it out on the diagram. It is often helpful for patients to understand why you might want them to transfer from one therapy to another. A typical example of this might be a patient who has used long-term beta-blockers with diazepam to control anxiety, whilst not using a drug like an SSRI or therapies such as CBT. Whilst using only medicines to control symptoms (i.e. the beta-blockers and benzodiazepines), these patients are not getting treatments to control the anxiety as a pathology.

Short circuit breakers

- CBT and other types of therapy
- 'Antidepressants'
    - e.g. SSRIs, SNRIs, TCAs, MAOIs.

Non-short circuit breakers

- Beta-blockers
    - relieve the adrenergic effects of anxiety but don't break the circuit
- Benzodiazepines
    - reduce agitation and induce calm but don't break the circuit
- Sleeping pills (e.g. zopiclone)
    - induce sleep but don't break the circuit.

Clearly there is a role for all medicines. When a patient is severely agitated or severely sleep-deprived, there may be a role for short-term symptom relief. However, after a patient is diagnosed with a long-term mental illness like anxiety or depression, the treatments offered should provide the patient with a safe long-term option that addresses pathology. Where you have used the short circuit tool, you can tell your patient that these interventions, if they work, will aim to break the short circuit, giving them relief of their symptoms in the longer term.

> ### Consultation tip - a note on 'happy pills'
>
> Antidepressants are commonly described by the public as 'happy pills'. I am usually very keen to tell my patients that this is not at all a good description of them. These medicines do not make people happy. Often people feel happy after taking them for a period of time. However, what is really happening is that the medicine is removing the pathology and the happy, smiling person that is revealed at the end was the real person. They were there all along, but hidden away under the mental health condition.
>
> This can be very effective in reassuring people that they are not somehow 'propped up' by chemicals and the 'real them' is simply revealed once the cloud of pathology is removed.

6.2 Treatment modalities

Treatment of a mental health condition in primary care can never be as protocolised as the treatment of asthma, diabetes or hypertension. In these fields one can recognise clear diagnostic tests, treatment targets and a stepwise approach to therapies. Conversely, treating a condition like depression or anxiety is a delicate balance of choosing the right treatment for the patient depending on a number of factors.

Earlier in the book, there was the separation of the three Ps – personality, pressure and pathology. This section is predominantly an exploration of the different treatment of pathology – from basic steps like exercise to combination drug augmentation strategies. However, as the patient's clinician, you will be asked to intervene on the 'pressure' element. This is dealt with in *Section 6.3: Dealing with pressure.*

Whilst it is of course useful to have a ladder of treatment modalities that you can progress up, it is more important to have a good mastery of all the interventions and treatments available for the patient. This will help you to choose and offer the best options for the patient in front of you. In reality there can never be a simple algorithm which tells you what to do for each mental health patient. The factors involved in your choice and offering to them are too diverse and personal to the individual in front of you.

6.2.1 List of common mental health treatments to understand and use

	General mental health	Sleep and agitation	Specific anxiety Rx
Key for all patients	Good education, advice and support	Sleep hygiene measures	
Low-end intervention	Watch, wait and review Sleep hygiene Mindfulness-based CBT Physical activity	Antihistamines	

Low-intensity intervention	Self-directed learning Computerised CBT Structured group exercise		
Higher-intensity	Medication: SSRIs, SNRIs, TCAs Mirtazapine, bupropion	Z-drugs Benzodiazepines	Beta-blockers
Highest level	Combination and augmentation MAOIs Antipsychotics		Pregabalin

6.2.2 General principles of treatment

Build a positive relationship

- Be open, develop trust and have a non-judgemental manner at all times.
- Instil hope and optimism – whilst the patient's past life will not change, the illnesses like depression can be treated and recovery is possible.
- Be aware of stigma. Patients may not wish to talk about mental health, it may have a negative or even offensive effect. Be mindful of this.
- Give information in an appropriate manner for the patient's understanding and ensure you have informed consent.
- Be respectful of, and sensitive to, diverse cultural, ethnic and religious backgrounds when working with people with mental health issues, and be aware of the possible variations in the presentation of these amongst different groups.

The following factors should also be taken into account when offering a treatment:

- Any history of mental illness and comorbid mental health or physical disorders
- Any past history of mood elevation (to determine if the depression may be part of bipolar disorder)
- Any past experience of, and response to, treatments
- The quality of interpersonal relationships

- Living conditions and social isolation
- The patient's beliefs and wishes.

In the following sections consideration is given to a number of different treatments, interventions and therapies. These generally go from low to high intensity; however, they should not be considered a simple 'one step follows another' treatment guide. Nevertheless, NICE does recommend a stepped-care model in which the least intrusive, most effective intervention and most tolerable intervention is offered first before moving upward.

NICE suggests the following factors that could help determine which level of intervention is necessary:

1. Factors that favour general advice and active monitoring:
   - Fewer symptoms with little associated disability
   - Symptoms intermittent, or of less than 2 weeks' duration
   - Recent onset with identified stressor
   - No past or family history of mental illness
   - Social support available
   - Lack of suicidal thoughts.
2. Factors that favour more active treatment in primary care:
   - More symptoms with higher associated disability
   - Persistent or long-standing symptoms
   - Personal or family history of mental illness
   - Low social support
   - Occasional suicidal thoughts.

6.2.3 General advice, support and education

All patients should have an appropriate assessment, support, education into the condition and active monitoring. Those deemed appropriate should be referred for further assessment and interventions.

It can be advisable, where appropriate and in partnership with the patient, to involve family or carers. You can advise a person with depression, for example, and their family or carer to be vigilant for mood changes, negativity and hopelessness, and suicidal ideation. They should be clear about who they should contact in times of concern – this would normally be their medical practitioner. This is particularly important during high-risk periods, such as starting or changing treatment and at times of increased personal stress.

6.2.4 Active monitoring – 'watch and wait'

Some people with low-level symptoms may recover with no formal intervention – you may wish to 'watch and wait'. You should, however, ensure that you:

- discuss the presenting problem(s) and any concerns that the person may have about them
- provide information about the nature and course of their illness
- arrange a further assessment – NICE recommends 2 weeks but you may wish to judge this with your patient
- make contact if the person does not attend follow-up appointments.

This is a perfectly reasonable strategy for patients with low-level symptoms. It can be useful if you feel there is not yet enough evidence to make a definitive diagnosis. Clearly this would not be appropriate for patients showing high levels of symptoms such as severe depression.

Pros:

- Simple intervention, not requiring any pharmacology or patient actions
- Could help reduce false positive diagnosis
- Gives patient and clinician more time to consider the diagnosis.

Cons:

- Can introduce a time delay to patients who need intervention.

6.2.5 Advice on sleep hygiene

Sleep disturbance is a common feature of many mental illnesses. There is good published literature to suggest that basic sleep hygiene methods can be useful. Patients can be directed to the NHS website which gives further information on good sleep hygiene[1]. A number of other online trusted resources are also available[2] [3]. Advice on sleep hygiene is also useful for patients without a recognised mental health diagnosis but who have a degree of insomnia.

General measures include:

- establishing regular sleep and wake times
- avoiding excess eating, smoking or drinking alcohol before sleep
- optimising the environment for sleep (online resources can help the patient achieve this)
- taking regular physical exercise.

Pros:

- Simple interventions which require no pharmacology
- Can help the patient feel empowered.

Cons:

- The patient may have already tried these things
- Limited efficacy beyond mild symptoms.

6.2.6 Exercise and physical activity

The condensed NICE guidelines 2009 do not include this recommendation; however, it is a commonly held belief that exercise can improve depression symptoms and some evidence does support this notion.

Overall, the evidence indicates that group-based physical activity is effective in the treatment of subthreshold and mild depression, when compared with no physical activity controls. For some people it can work as well as SSRIs in the subthreshold group; however, it must be stressed that exercise alone will likely be insufficient to treat patients with higher levels of depression.

The research is unclear over how long the exercise needs to be done for, or how intensely, before depression symptoms begin to reduce. Theories on the reason that exercise improves depres-

---

[1] www.nhs.uk/live-well/sleep-and-tiredness/how-to-get-to-sleep/
[2] www.sleepfoundation.org/sleep-hygiene
[3] https://sleepeducation.org/healthy-sleep/healthy-sleep-habits/

sion vary. Whilst high-intensity exercise can release endorphins, producing a short-lived improvement in mood, it's likely that low-intensity exercise sustained over time can improve nerve cell growth and connections.

Even without the evidence that exercise improves depression, it is clearly an important message for all patients for a variety of other health reasons. Exercising produces a cascade of physiological effects that results in many health benefits, such as protecting against heart disease and diabetes, improving sleep and lowering blood pressure.

Pros:

- Many other health benefits
- Can help the patient feel empowered
- No 'drugs' involved.

Cons:

- Uptake can be limited
- Less suitable for people with physical disability
- Evidence is supportive for lowest levels of depression only.

6.2.7 Mindfulness-based cognitive therapy (MBCT)

Clinical results suggest that mindfulness-based therapy is a promising intervention for treating anxiety and mood problems in clinical populations. Mindfulness is recommended by NICE as a way to prevent relapse of depression symptoms. This is a mental training technique that encourages awareness of thoughts, feelings, moods and bodily sensations as they are in the present moment.

By paying attention to these thoughts and feelings right now, the patient is able to become better at spotting the build-up of difficult emotions and thoughts and can deal with them more skilfully, instead of just reacting in ways that may worsen the situation.

Mindfulness practices include focusing on the breath and body as well as mindful movement, and developing greater mindful attention to everyday activities. Mindfulness focuses the mind on normally ignored sensations, such as the touch of clothes on the skin or the feeling of gravity pulling the body into a chair.

Mindfulness can be practised in group sessions or alone, and a number of different phone apps, web-based services and local group services are available.

Pros:

- Can be very tolerable to most people and only requires a short time per day to use
- No 'drugs' involved
- Can be learned and used when needed in the future.

Cons:

- Some services require a paid subscription
- Doesn't work for everyone.

6.3 Dealing with pressure

In *Section 2.4*, I introduced the separation of person, pressure and pathology. The primary purpose of this is to reassure the patient that their mental health condition is distinct from their own sense of self. It helps them see that a diagnosis such as depression or anxiety is not a reflection on their personality, nor a reflection on their ability to cope with life pressures.

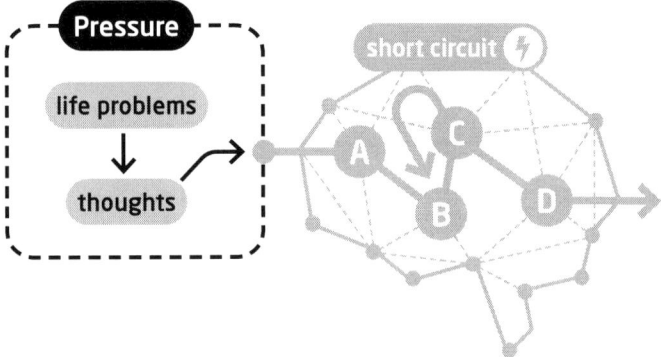

Nevertheless, using the short circuit tool, it is clear that patients with both pathology and high levels of pressure will be suffering the most. Where pathology is present, thoughts will bounce from B to C to B. But the nature, severity and quality of the troubling thoughts are also proportional to the life pressure that the individual is under.

Whilst much of this book is targeted toward the clinician's response to the presence of pathology in the patient, it is often also the case that the clinician may be able to help with lightening the pressure load too. At first glance, it can seem that some of the life pressures that an individual is under are completely outside of the influence of their doctor, and in some cases that may be true.

The complex socioeconomic and personal circumstances that any individual can find themselves in are almost infinitely varied and the factors that contribute to this are equally varied. These will all have an influence on the mental and physical wellbeing of the individual. It is also a common occurrence that the individual will look to their healthcare provider for some help with their personal circumstances.

In light of this, it is vitally important that the clinician both understands and appreciates the patient's individual circumstances but also has an understanding of where they can influence these, or at least what tools are available for them to influence. This has been an area of significant research in recent years under the banner of 'wider determinants of health'. Public Heath England provides significant tools and resources to explore further. [4]

Consider the following interventions:

6.3.1 Fit notes

Fit notes are well-recognised by the medical profession and, at the time of writing, can only be issued by a doctor. It is outside the scope of this book to analyse the use of fit notes in detail, but they can be used in a mental health setting to influence the quantum of pressure that a patient is under.

The fit note can be a key tool for you to use to improve your patient's health and be an advocate for their wellbeing. A note which allows the patient time off work to recover is naturally beneficial. This can be for the obvious reason that the patient's health makes it impossible or difficult to conduct their work. However, on occasion, the patient's workplace can be the principal site of stress and life pressure, and the use of the fit note to relieve this can be invaluable.

[4] https://fingertips.phe.org.uk/profile/wider-determinants

Research suggests patients are generally happy for their GP to give them advice on work issues, and do not feel that this threatens the doctor–patient relationship [5].

Work is generally beneficial for health, both mental and physical. Therefore the fit note should fundamentally play a role in helping patients return to work as soon as is appropriate and feasible. Patients do not have to be 100% fit in order to work, in most cases. The fit note supports people to work when they can and gives them an option to amend duties and work hours if this is better than being off work altogether. There is, therefore, a 'sweet spot' of length of time off work, particularly for mental health conditions. This will naturally vary between patients, depending on the severity of illness.

The longer a patient is off work, the lower their chances are of making a successful return to work; this important and well-evidenced fact should be borne in mind the longer a patient is off work. You should counsel a patient who has been off for an extended period that their return to normality (including a return to work) can be considered a tool in their rehabilitation from a mental illness.

The Department of Work and Pensions has produced an excellent document entitled *Getting the most out of your fit note*, in collaboration with the BMA, ACAS and RCGP, and this is good reading for any GP using fit notes in their practice. [6]

6.3.2 Letters and reports

From time to time, particularly as the patient's GP, you will be asked for letters, reports and statements to assist the patient in terms of their housing, employment, social circumstances or other needs.

---

[5] O'Brien, K., Cadbury, N., Rollnick, S. and Wood, F. (2008) Sickness certification in the general practice consultation: the patients' perspective, a qualitative study. *Fam Pract.*, **25(1):** 20–6.

[6] https://assets.publishing.service.gov.uk/government/uploads/system/uploads/attachment_data/file/298821/fitnote-gps-guidance-jan-14.pdf

For the most part, these requests are not covered under the remit of the NHS and the GMS GP contract in the UK and will therefore often carry a charge to the patient or those that have requested the report. It is, again, outside the remit of this book to detail the vast possibilities of what you can or can't, and should or should not do.

Nevertheless, there are circumstances in which a relatively simple intervention from a clinician can have a significant impact on the stress and life pressure levels that a patient is undergoing.

Remember that a patient is entitled to a copy of their own medical record free of charge under GDPR rules. If a patient simply needs a copy of their notes to prove a condition or treatment to their employer or another agency, then they are entitled to it and there should not be a charge. When a patient is finding it difficult to pay for a full report, you should consider whether a simple print-off of their notes or a summary of their notes would perform the job they are after. Increasingly, patients have digital access to their own notes and this can do the same job.

Where a clinician's opinion is required or a specific report is asked for, there is likely to be a fee to pay. In many circumstances the patient becomes the 'middle man' between the agency wanting a report and the doctor writing the report. Sometimes the report or letter you write doesn't contain the information that the agency requires, meaning that there is further contact and writing.

When a patient has come asking for such a report, it may be advisable to tell the patient to ask the agency or employer to write to the practice directly. This will allow them to ask exactly what they need and the practice can be transparent about the fees it will charge and to whom.

When a patient is suffering from a mental health condition and they are put in a position of chasing letters and reports, this can significantly add to their stress levels. It is important to recognise this and try to help the patient out of their predicament.

6.3.3 Social prescribing

Social prescribing is not a new concept but has been given a significant boost in availability to patients and clinicians and forms a key component of 'Universal Personalised Care', a policy favoured by NHS England to give people more choice and control over their own mental and physical healthcare. [7]

Clinicians in primary care are often taught that their patient's condition is the result of a complex biopsychosocial mesh. However, they are often only equipped to deal with the patient's biological pathology. This leaves the psychosocial aspect unaddressed. Addressing this requires time, resources, an intricate knowledge of local services and the ability to follow the patient up at regular intervals. Many clinicians would love to have the time to do this but in an environment with many competing demands, they often are not able to.

There is a growing body of evidence which shows that social prescribing improves wellbeing for people. Evaluations of local social prescribing schemes have reported reduced pressure on NHS services, with reductions in GP consultations, A&E attendances and hospital bed stays. In 2017, the University of Westminster published an Evidence Summary[8], which identified 28% fewer GP consultations and 24% fewer A&E attendances for people receiving social prescribing support. An evaluation of a social prescribing project in Bristol from the early 2010s [9] highlighted improvements in anxiety levels and in feelings about general health and quality of life. Analysis by the RCGP found that social prescribing was among the most effective of the ten high-impact actions at reducing GP workload. [10]

---

[7] www.england.nhs.uk/personalisedcare/upc/

[8] Polley, M.J., Fleming, J., Anfilogoff, T. and Carpenter, A. (2017) *Making Sense of Social Prescribing*. University of Westminster.

[9] Kimberlee, R.H. (2013) *Developing a Social Prescribing Approach for Bristol*. University of the West of England.

[10] www.rcgp.org.uk/policy/general-practice-forward-view.aspx (click on the "Spotlight on the 10 High Impact Actions" link)

Whilst social prescribing is still not universally available to all primary care clinicians, its reach is ever-expanding. Where it is available, there is an individual called the 'link worker' to whom the patient can be referred. The link worker can then consult with the patient and begin to address the wider determinants of the individual's health. Link workers give people time, focusing on 'what matters to me' and taking a holistic approach to people's health and wellbeing. In the short circuit analogy for patients with a mental health condition, this addresses the second P – pressure.

For the most part, patients who can be referred to a link worker are those:

- with one or more long-term conditions
- who need support with their mental health
- who are lonely or isolated
- who have complex social needs which affect their wellbeing.

Whilst social prescribing has been developed with primary care and general practice in mind, it can and should be accessible to a wide range of agencies. The emphasis on the availability to general practice was simply a logistical one, in that many people will still see their own GP as a primary port of call for health issues which have a social causative element. Other agencies which should be able to refer into social prescribing (i.e. to a link worker) include (but are not limited to):

- pharmacies
- multidisciplinary teams
- hospital discharge teams
- allied health professionals
- fire service and police
- job centres
- social care services
- housing associations and voluntary, community and social enterprise (VCSE) organisations.

Self-referral is also encouraged.

Once the patient has been referred to the link worker, they can start a number of interventions. Link workers are recruited for their listening skills, empathy and ability to support people. On average, link workers have between six and twelve contacts with a person, depending on their needs, over a 3-month period. Other terms for the same role include community connector, wellbeing advisor, community navigator and health advisor, depending on local preference.

Once the patient is known to the link worker they can be offered a range of different services and interventions, depending on the locally available services. The voluntary sector is often fundamental to the provision of many of these services. Examples of these include:

- Physical activities
  - gyms and exercise classes
  - weight management and nutrition
- Arts-based activities
- Employment-based and volunteering activities
- Support to access welfare rights
- Debt and housing advice, and advocacy services.

Social prescribing is a much-needed tool in the armoury in the fight against mental illness. Where it is available, you should be aware of it and use it. At the time of writing, about 75% of GP practices have access to a social prescriber. The evidence is strongly in favour of improved outcomes in your patient and a reduction in resource burden on the NHS and general practice.

6.4 Cognitive behavioural therapy

Cognitive behavioural therapy (CBT) is an important instrument for the treatment of mental health problems. It is a psychosocial intervention that is well-evidenced in improving a range of mental health conditions. CBT relies on the assumption that by changing thinking (cognition) and behaviour, an individual can indirectly influence mood and affect, thereby treating a number of mental health disorders such as depression, anxiety, post-traumatic stress disorder, substance abuse, eating disorders and borderline personality disorder, amongst others. CBT can be practised by primary care clinicians in the 10-minute consultation and an excellent guide is *Using CBT in General Practice* by Dr Lee David.[11]

Using the short circuit tool, *Section 6.3* focused on the second P, pressure. CBT on the other hand addresses the third P, pathology. This is the short circuit and by breaking it, the pathology is improved.

CBT focuses on challenging and changing unhelpful cognition (e.g. thoughts, beliefs and attitudes) and behaviours, improving emotional regulation, and the development of personal coping strategies that target solving current problems.

It is fundamentally different to other psychotherapy techniques such as the more historical psychoanalysis, where the therapist looks for the unconscious meaning behind the behaviours and then formulates a diagnosis. In contrast, CBT is a 'problem-focused' and 'action-oriented' form of therapy and does not usually involve a deep exploration of a person's history such as their childhood or past relationships (unless this is specifically indicated for that individual).

It is fundamentally important, as a clinician referring a patient to a CBT service, to explain the 'problem and action' focus. It is often the case that the patient's preconception of what they are being referred for is that of psychoanalytical psychotherapy, which is a very different technique. This basic explanation could be instrumental in determining the patient's engagement with the service.

---

[11]   David, L. (2013) *Using CBT in General Practice*, second edition. Scion Publishing Ltd.

6.4.1 A brief history

The modern-day notion of CBT has a strong correlation with the ancient philosophy of stoicism, first described in ancient Greece in the 3rd century BC. Stoic philosophers believed logic could be used to identify and discard false beliefs that lead to destructive emotions.

Modern CBT started with the development of behaviour therapy in the 1920s, followed by cognitive therapy in the 1960s (developed largely by Aaron Beck), which later merged to become cognitive behavioural theory in the 1980s–90s. Originally it was designed to treat depression, but its uses have been expanded to include treatment of a number of mental health conditions. Over time, cognitive behavioural therapy came to be known not only as a therapy, but as an umbrella term for a number of related cognitive-based psychotherapies.

6.4.2 Evidence base

CBT is well-evidenced overall, showing the highest affinity for success in major depression and anxiety disorders. Studies have shown that cognitive therapy is as efficacious as antidepressant medications at treating depression, and it seems to reduce the risk of relapse even after its discontinuation. There are studies, however, that suggest that one or the other is better. A major criticism of clinical studies of CBT efficacy (or any psychotherapy) has been that they are not double-blind. Double-blinding is extremely difficult to achieve in this field.

Some research suggests that CBT is most effective when combined with medication for treating major depressive disorder. However, other research has suggested the two approaches yield equal results – particularly at the lower end of the severity spectrum.

NICE has recommended CBT as the gold standard form of psychotherapy for a number of decades and it forms part of the stepped therapy guidelines for depression, anxiety and a number of other common mental health disorders.

6.4.3 How does CBT work?

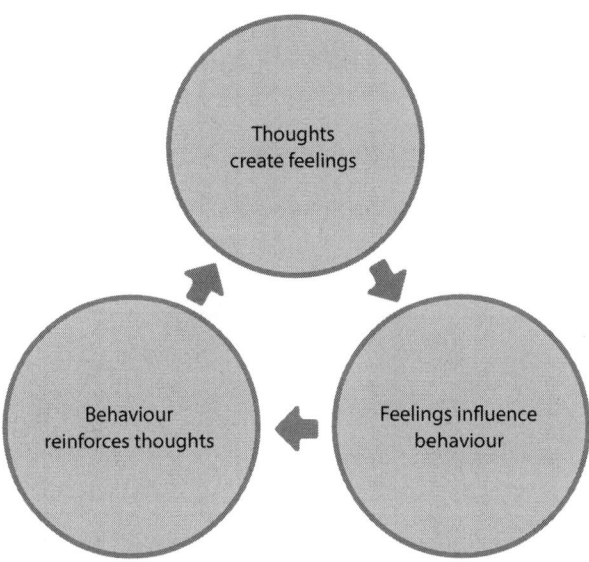

CBT is based on the idea that thinking (cognition), feeling (emotion) and action (behaviour) interact together, having a significant influence on each other. Thoughts determine feelings, feelings determine behaviour and behaviour in turn determines thoughts. Influencing parts of the cycle that are more easily and directly controlled – such as behaviours – will, in turn, have an effect on the others. Mental health is a function of feelings, emotion and thoughts, so this technique is well-suited to the treatment of mental illness.

Therefore, negative and unrealistic thoughts can cause distress and result in illness. When a patient suffers with psychological distress, the way in which they interpret situations becomes skewed, which in turn has a negative impact on the actions they take.

CBT aims to help patients become aware of when they make negative interpretations, and of behavioural patterns which reinforce this thinking. CBT's intended effect is to develop alternative ways of thinking and behaving which aim to reduce the psychological distress.

Case study - Peter

Peter is a 40-year-old accounts clerk with a young family. Peter has lived with mild anxiety for several years, but recently it's become worse. His anxious thoughts mainly relate to conditions at his workplace.

Recently, after the company showed signs of a financial downturn, Peter has become worried about the loss of his job and he feels his co-workers may be targeting him for redundancy.

Peter's co-workers continue to be friendly and his manager seems to be happy with his performance; however, Peter can't stop worrying that others dislike him and that he will suddenly lose his job. He replays scenarios in his head over and over about the negative impact of this on his young family.

Peter particularly finds certain scenarios distressing – including being in a meeting with several people or being in the social room taking lunch with others in the room. He has, for the last 4 months, started to avoid these as much as possible.

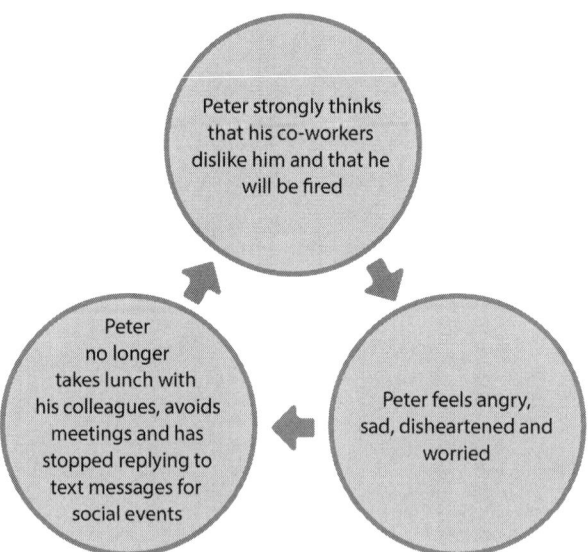

In this example, it can be seen that Peter's behaviours and action choices further exacerbate his way of thinking, which further entrenches his feeling of anxiety.

The cognitive behavioural therapist has a number of techniques to challenge and change Peter's outlook, including (but not limited to):

- **Cognitive restructuring or reframing**
  - this involves looking at negative thought patterns and attempting to alter them, such as not over-generalising, assuming the worst outcome or over-valuing a minor detail
- **Guided discovery**
  - the therapist will acquaint themselves with the patient's viewpoint; they'll then ask questions to challenge the patient's beliefs and broaden their thinking
  - this could involve being asked to give evidence that supports the assumptions about why the patient is thinking is a certain way
- **Exposure therapy**
  - this can be used to help desensitise the patient to scenarios and places that cause certain emotions and physical responses
  - in Peter's case this might include starting to attend more meetings and engage with lunchtime conversation
- **Journaling and thought records**
  - the therapist will ask Peter to write down both positive and negative thoughts and feelings; this has the effect of helping the patient get in touch with their own thoughts
- **Behavioural experiments**
  - this can be useful for anxiety problems that lead to catastrophic thinking. The therapist may ask Peter to 'predict' what will happen in certain scenarios (such as attending a meeting). Over time the fact that the predicted catastrophe does not happen will challenge the thought process
- **Relaxation and stress reduction techniques**
  - these include deep breathing, muscle relaxation and imagery; these techniques are strongly associated with mindfulness and meditation

- **Role playing**
  - the therapist may play out scenarios, helping to improve problem-solving skills, improving confidence and social interaction skills.

6.4.4 Ways to access cognitive behavioural therapy

The type of CBT offered to your patient will of course depend on the availability of services in the area, although the national standard is such that all patients should be able to access CBT. The patient's own attitude towards this should also be considered, as well as any previous attempts.

- Has the patient seen a CBT practitioner previously?
- What was the outcome?
- Why did it/didn't it work?
- Ability to engage (time factors, work factors)
- Relationship with practitioner – does the patient prefer computer-based or human interaction?

Low-intensity CBT

NICE describes the following as 'low intensity' CBT packages:

Individual guided self-help based on the principles of CBT

For guided self-help, the patient will be doing much of the reading but will have some structured support from a mentor. The professional involved in the mentoring may not, however, have the same level of training as a fully qualified CBT practitioner.

NICE recommends that if this is offered, individual guided self-help programmes should include the provision of written materials of an appropriate reading age and be supported by a trained practitioner, who typically facilitates the self-help programme and reviews progress and outcome. It usually consists of up to six to eight sessions (face-to-face or via telephone) and normally takes place over 9–12 weeks, including follow-up.

Computerised cognitive behavioural therapy (CCBT)

CCBT has been described by NICE as a "generic term for delivering CBT via an interactive computer interface delivered by a personal computer, internet, or interactive voice response system instead of face-to-face with a human therapist".

The main advantage of CCBT was to overcome the costs and lack of availability of human therapists and improve access for patients with limited time to dedicate to the process. It has been shown in trials to be cost-effective.

However, other studies have shown that CCBT suffers from low uptake after a clinician has referred, and completion rates are low in those who have started. Low-intensity CBT is also associated with a higher rate of relapse in patients who do successfully complete it. NICE does not endorse any specific product.

A current focus of research is in the combination of artificial intelligence and CCBT to improve its individual impact on the patient.

Pros:

- May be more accessible to some patients with work commitments
- Model has great appeal because it focuses on human thought and can feel empowering
- Not 'drug-based' and this will suit certain individuals
- Techniques can be remembered and used again in the future.

Cons:

- Evidence suggests lower rates of engagement and completion compared to high-intensity therapy
- Relies heavily on patient motivation
- May not suit patients with learning difficulty
- Higher rate of relapse in contrast to high-intensity therapy
- Local services may be lacking if not specifically commissioned
- Evidence holds for low-severity levels of anxiety and depression only.

High-intensity CBT

One-to-one therapy with a CBT practitioner is usually described as 'high-intensity' CBT. A typical CBT programme would consist of face-to-face sessions between patient and therapist, made up of 12–15 sessions of around an hour each, with a gap of 1–3 weeks between sessions. This number is flexible and there will be cases that need more and those that need fewer sessions. The client and practitioner will normally agree this together.

CBT is associated with the 'scientist–practitioner' model. This usually includes clear defining of the problem, an emphasis on measurement, including measuring changes in cognition and behaviour and in the attainment of goals.

Often therapists will give 'homework' assignments in which the patient and the therapist work together to craft an assignment to complete before the next session. The completion of these homework tasks – which can be as simple as a person suffering from anxiety attending some kind of social event – indicates a dedication to treatment compliance and a desire to change. The therapist can then decide the next step of treatment based on how thoroughly the patient completes the assignment. A therapeutic alliance between the therapist and the patient is essential in achieving a good outcome. The patient is therefore very involved in high-intensity CBT and 'completing the homework' forms an essential part of the therapy.

If that is achieved, the therapy can move on but if not, the patient and therapist must work together to reassign the goal. Flexibility and willingness to listen to the patient, rather than acting as an authority figure, are essential features of a good therapist.

Pros:

- Much more tailored to the individual patient
- Ability to measure changes and document progress more scientifically
- Not 'drug-based' and this will suit certain individuals
- Techniques can be remembered and used again in the future
- Evidence is supportive of this approach even for high levels of illness severity.

Cons:

- Relies heavily on patient motivation and requires time commitment at specific hours
- May not suit patients with learning difficulty
- The precise role of cognitive processes is yet to be determined. It is not clear whether faulty cognitions are a cause of the psychopathology or a consequence of it. This can confuse some patients
- Services are normally commissioned throughout the country but waiting times can be long.

6.5 Pharmacological treatments

There are of course many different drug treatments available for a range of mental health conditions; the subsections below cover these in order, very roughly, from 'weakest' to 'strongest'. Each works in its own unique way and has its own characteristics. Unfortunately many of these are talked about in the same single category of 'antidepressants'.

The term antidepressant can be unhelpful if used too generically without reference to the type in question. In the first instance the term is used to describe a number of quite different drug categories. Also, the so-called 'antidepressant' is equally effective in a range of mental health conditions other than depression. Calling these drugs antidepressants does little to inform, educate and empower the patient to understand what they are being treated for and how their treatments are working. Of course the term is widely recognised and used by the general public and in the medical profession so its use cannot be avoided. However, explaining the specific type of medicine that the patient is using is often helpful.

The single most ubiquitous 'antidepressant' is the SSRI. This class of drug is recommended by NICE as the treatment of choice and at the time of writing there does not appear to be any other drug on the horizon that will match its flexibility and usefulness.

In relation to the short circuit tool, all so-called 'antidepressants' effectively aim to break the circuit and therefore, as interventions, can be helpful in a number of mental health disorders.

6.5.1 Herbal

St John's wort

Whilst there are some studies which suggest a benefit to the use of St John's wort (*Hypericum perforatum*), there is little concrete evidence.

It is sold ubiquitously in chemists, health food shops and online and is used by many individuals. It should not be prescribed and is not recommended for depression by NICE. St John's wort is a potential metabolising enzyme inducer and therefore has a number of important interactions with other drugs, including commonly used antidepressant drugs such as SSRIs and SNRIs. The amount of active ingredient can vary hugely between different preparations of St John's wort and switching from one to another can change the degree of enzyme induction.

As a metabolising enzyme inducer, St John's wort will reduce the active concentration of the other medication. Therefore, when a patient stops taking St John's wort, the concentration of the interacting drugs may increase, leading to toxicity.

6.5.2 SSRIs

A brief history

In the 1980s, a class of drugs called selective serotonin reuptake inhibitors (SSRIs) emerged on the market. These were considered, at the time, a medical science breakthrough. Eli Lilly, the company that brought Prozac (fluoxetine) to the mass market, started in 1971 with a compound known as LY110141. It intended this to be a treatment for high blood pressure. The substance seemed to work in animals but they had a hard time getting the same results in humans. Giving up on this, the researchers tried to see if they could get it to work as an anti-obesity drug. Again, no luck. Eventually they tried it on patients with depression. At the more extreme end of the spectrum the patients did not improve but those with moderate symptoms showed huge improvements in their depressive symptoms. Realising the potential to market this new medicine, Eli Lilly wanted to push this new marvel drug hard. This was the first time that a medicine for depression was given the same marketing as Coca Cola, Nike or Sony and it was an international hit. It promised to be bliss in a blister pack and was dubbed 'the happy pill'. Promoted to the world through celebrities, expensive adverts and through campaigning on the dangers of depression directly to the public, Prozac itself has earned its parent company billions. Of course, this dubious blurring of the lines between medical altruism and cold hard product promotion has led many to be suspicious.

It's hardly surprising then, that the average man or woman in the street would hold a generally negative view of drugs. Is it really worth trying to treat a condition with a chemical that might cause you serious harm, that could have you addicted or is out there being pushed by a big drug company earning billions from it?

You may find that as a clinician you have to overcome this and many other stereotypes to present a clear and rational offer to your patient.

Current SSRIs

These are the SSRIs currently readily available for prescribing:

- Citalopram
- Escitalopram
- Fluoxetine
- Fluvoxamine
- Paroxetine
- Sertraline
- Vortioxetine.

How to choose an SSRI

A recent meta-analysis conducted in 2018 [12] found virtually no difference in efficacy between the different SSRIs. There are, however, some subtle and important differences in the duration of action of these medicines which may help you choose.

Fluoxetine has a longer half-life and is therefore associated with fewer discontinuation syndrome effects. Paroxetine, on the other hand, is more strongly associated with discontinuation syndrome

---

[12] Cipriani, A., Furukawa, T., Salanti, G. *et al.* (2018) Comparative efficacy and acceptability of 21 antidepressant drugs for the acute treatment of adults with major depressive disorder: a systematic review and network meta-analysis. *Lancet*, **391(10128):** 1357–1366.

since it has the shortest half-life. Paroxetine is also being reported to have a higher likelihood of toxicity and interaction with other medicines. For this reason it's probably now considered the least appropriate SSRI.

As for the others, there seems to be little to choose between them. Side-effect profiles and overall clinical effectiveness are roughly equal. Your choice and offering to the patient should be of an SSRI that you are comfortable with and which is cost-effective and prescribed in a generic form. The only exception is vortioxetine which is a more recently released and approved drug which may be more effective. Vortioxetine has been the subject of a separate 2015 NICE technology appraisal[13].

There is no value whatsoever in prescribing a certain SSRI based on the patient demographic such as age or sex. These associations have been studied and found not to hold any value in helping you to prescribe.

Starting an SSRI

If and when you start an SSRI for your patient it is vitally important that you don't just give them a prescription. There are a number of significant things that you must explain to the patient. Failure to do this will dramatically increase the chance of a drop in compliance and a failure to achieve the therapeutic benefit of the drug.

NICE provides a list of five things that should be covered in the initial consultation, aside from the obvious important patient consultation issues such as exploring concerns the person has about taking medication and explaining fully the reasons for prescribing. It suggests providing the following pieces of information about taking antidepressants:

- The gradual development of the full antidepressant effect – this will take weeks
- The importance of taking medication as prescribed and the need to continue treatment after remission
- Potential side-effects

---

[13] NICE (2015) *Vortioxetine for treating major depressive episodes.* Technology appraisal guidance [TA367].

- The nature of discontinuation symptoms with all antidepressants and how these symptoms can be minimised
- The fact that addiction does not occur with antidepressants.

Whilst it is, of course, natural to have these discussions with any patient about any treatment, I strongly believe that in the treatment of mental health this becomes of paramount importance.

Fear and nocebo

It is, for very clear and obvious reasons, well understood and accepted that a clinician treating a patient for any condition should give a full and frank disclosure of the nature of the treatment given. This should, of course, include a breakdown of the intended benefits and – of equal importance – a clear picture of possible harmful side-effects or complications.

A surgeon obtaining a patient's consent would not be reassured that the consent was valid without a documented conversation with the patient about what the possible unintended sequelae were. The validity of consent is complex and outside the sphere of this book to cover, but one of the basic tenets is that the patient must be given all the material information in terms of what the treatment involves, including the benefits and risks, whether there are reasonable alternative treatments, and what will happen if treatment doesn't go ahead.

It would be wholly irresponsible and unacceptable to assume that you can start any course of treatment, whether pharmacological or talking-based, without a discussion on side-effects. However, there is a layer of practicality. No clinician will relay the whole *BNF* entry to their patient, for fairly self-evident reasons. You often have a short time to get across the key, important facts.

Nevertheless, the way in which these are discussed is very important. The language used, the key facts chosen to disclose, the examples given and the expectations suggested can be pivotal. It should also be noted that patients will already have a great deal of preconception about 'antidepressants' – more so than other medicines – which will be informing their view and expectation of their action.

As clinicians we are well versed in the concept of the placebo effect. Less is heard in general parlance about the nocebo effect. This is the symmetrical opposite of the placebo: it is a negative side-effect that is experienced by a person taking an inert substance whose expectations are such that they are likely to feel unwell as a result. Just as the interpersonal and environmental dimensions of the clinical encounter have a potentially powerful therapeutic benefit (placebo), negative aspects of the clinical encounter can have negative, nocebo effects.

Fascinatingly, there are well-documented instances of patients in the placebo arm getting side-effects that exactly match those listed as side-effects of the active drug. For example, when the placebo arm of a tricyclic drug trial was compared with the placebo arm of an SSRI drug trial, patients receiving TCA placebos reported higher rates than those receiving SSRI placebos of dry mouth (19.2% vs. 6.4%), vision problems (6.9% vs. 1.2%), fatigue (17.3% vs. 5.5%) and constipation (10.7% vs. 4.2%) [14]. Both sets of patients received a completely inert substance. However, those patients who believed they may be taking the tricyclic had very significantly higher rates of tricyclic-like side-effects.

The skill of the clinician is to provide the patient with a clear, honest and helpful picture of the treatment that they are giving, without eliciting an unnecessary nocebo effect.

Five key messages

1 Time to onset

Always tell your patient that these medicines will take several weeks or even up to a month to work. Many patients will expect some degree of improvement with a medicine well before then if they have not been counselled on this. Patients can feel demoralised when their medicines have failed to make any difference. This can especially be the case when the patient has waited a long time to see the doctor and built up significant courage in accepting a diagnosis or starting a treatment. It may even have the effect

---

[14]   Colloca, L. and Miller, F.G. (2011) The nocebo effect and its relevance for clinical practice. *Psychosom Med.*, **73(7):** 598–603.

of worsening a person's mental health condition when they feel that treatments are not working.

This is also commonly seen when patients have tried several different medicines for a short time, believing that each one has not worked. I hear patients tell me many times that they have tried antidepressants in the past without success. On examination of the notes I sometimes find that they have been on the medication for 4 weeks or under. Clearly this would not have been long enough for the medicine to have been fully evaluated, but it can leave a lasting impression on the patient that this form of therapy will not work for them.

2 The drug is not addictive

No research trial has found SSRIs to be addictive. NICE makes it clear in its guidance that clinicians should counsel specifically on this fact. Nevertheless many websites, social media outlets and newspapers – both tabloid and broadsheet – will argue the opposite. The medical profession should show a degree of humility in accepting that the research thus far may end up being wrong. Nevertheless it is clearly accepted that fair and detailed research trials will produce a more accurate result than anecdote and mass media articles.

For many patients, getting this knowledge can be incredibly powerful. Often the single most important factor in people rejecting treatments for depression or anxiety is the belief that the medicines will be addictive. Often the relief in people's minds can be quite palpable. In fact many patients who have been on these drugs for a long period of time lived with a degree of fear and guilt that the drug they take will be causing them harm in the long run. If you, as the patient's clinician, can assure them that these drugs are not addictive, it will likely have an immediate relieving and lifting effect.

> No research trial has found SSRIs to be addictive. NICE makes it clear in its guidance that clinicians should counsel specifically on this fact.

3 Side-effects

It is of course important to explain to the patient that they may get some side-effects. In my consultations this is often the second question asked when we start talking about SSRIs – the first question being 'are they addictive?'.

Rather than reeling off a multitude of possible side-effects and scaring the patients, you could direct them to the NHS website www.nhs.uk which gives a good summary of what to expect.

In my consultations, I often use the following as an explanation for the patient.

- First, the majority of patients (over 50–60%) will experience no or very mild side-effects. These will be no more than effects that they may notice but which should not cause any major concern or trouble.
- About 30–40% of patients will get some degree of side-effect which could cause some distress. The most common of these are gastric side-effects such as bloating or feeling sick, feeling agitated, shaky or anxious, blurred vision, unusual dreams and sexual side-effects such as difficulty in achieving orgasm. The symptoms are likely to be much more pronounced in the first few weeks and are very likely to subside.
- A further 10% of patients may experience more significant side-effects to the extent that they will find it difficult to tolerate the medicine. I ask such patients to contact me at the surgery. Few patients will be in this group; however, it's important to explain that this could be the case for any patient, as it's difficult to predict what side-effects any one individual will get.

Most of these side-effects are short-term, especially during the initiation phase; however, there are others which are more likely to affect patients in the long term. The single most common of these are the sexual dysfunction side-effects such as lowered libido and inability to achieve orgasm. Some patients have noted a weight gain effect and some sleep disturbance. However, these effects can be sporadic and quite variable between patients. Side-effects that can occur include:

- feeling agitated, shaky or anxious
- nausea
- dizziness or blurred vision
- low sex drive, difficulty achieving orgasm and erectile dysfunction

- in some cases, an increase in thoughts of self-harm and suicidal ideation has been reported in the initial few weeks of initiation of an SSRI (particularly in young patients).

SSRIs and suicide risk

In May 2003, an SSRI expert working group[15] was established to consider the safety of SSRIs, including the issue of suicidal risk. The group reviewed all available data and concluded the following:

- Generally in depressed patients the risk of suicide is greatest around the time of their presentation to medical services; however, the risk of suicide may increase in the early stages of treatment for depressive illness
- A modest increase in the risk of suicidal thoughts and self-harm for SSRIs compared with placebo cannot be ruled out
- There is insufficient evidence of any marked difference in suicidal risk between the different SSRIs, or between SSRIs and other antidepressants.

SSRIs and mania

In the presence of bipolar disorder, SSRIs, when given without the combination with a mood stabiliser, can induce a hypomanic state. In patients with known bipolar disorder who are not on any psychiatric medicines, and who present with a depressive episode, SSRIs alone should not be used without consultation with a secondary care clinician.

Serotonin syndrome

Serotonin syndrome is extremely rare but is potentially serious. It is associated with SSRIs, when used in the presence of multiple serotonergic drugs such as tramadol, tricyclics, lithium, carbamazepine and others. MAO inhibitors have a particularly high associated risk.

Symptoms can include very high fever, confusion, agitation, muscle twitching, sweating, diarrhoea and tachycardia.

The diagnosis is clinical and a strong suspicion should result in immediate assessment in an acute hospital.

---

[15] Weller, I.V.D., Ashby, D., Brook, R. *et al.* (2005) *Report of the CSM Expert Working Group on the safety of selective serotonin reuptake inhibitor antidepressants.* MHRA.

4 Discontinuation effect

Whilst many SSRIs can be associated with initiation effects as described above, they can also be associated with discontinuation effects. It is extremely important to understand that this is fundamentally different to addiction, withdrawal and tolerance. The discontinuation syndrome is defined as a set of side-effects that occur when the drug is stopped. The symptoms associated with this can include (but are not limited to):

- restlessness
- trouble sleeping
- unsteadiness
- sweating
- stomach problems
- feeling as if there's an electric shock in your head
- feeling irritable, anxious or confused.

For the majority of patients these symptoms are extremely mild or even non-existent. They can start within a few days of stopping the medicine and last for several weeks afterwards. They can look as if the patient is addicted to the medicine and is withdrawing.

In fact medication discontinuation effects are extremely common across a range of different medicines, including steroid inhalers and beta-blockers.

The chances of these effects occurring can be minimised by reducing the dose and withdrawing the SSRI over a number of weeks; NICE recommends about 4 weeks. However, this may vary between patients. This is in stark contrast to the withdrawal of a truly addictive medicine such as a benzodiazepine or an opioid, which can take many months or even years to completely remove from the body and would be associated with cravings for the drug.

The SSRI paroxetine is most associated with this effect and for this reason is often not used. Due to the long half-life of fluoxetine (see table) it is least associated with the discontinuation effect.

Explain to your patient that they may get side-effects when they first start the medicine for the first few weeks and they may get side-effects when they stop the medicine for the first few weeks.

Drug	Half-life (hours)
Paroxetine	21
Escitalopram	29.5
Citalopram	25
Sertraline	83
Fluoxetine	240

5 Duration of taking the medicine

Finally, I think it's very important to get across to the patient the likely duration of them being on the medicine. Many patients naturally assume that they will be on a short course of pills. In fact the minimum recommended duration of taking an SSRI is 6 months; for the majority of patients it's going to be longer. For patients who have had a relapse of depression or anxiety, the accepted advice is 2 years. Some patients with multiple relapses may benefit from staying on the drug for many years. The drug is not associated with long-term physiological harm to the body.

It's important to counsel patients not to stop their medicine when they're feeling better. Often the effects kick in after a number of weeks and without this advice many patients will stop the medicine.

Patients will naturally want to know if they will be on it lifelong. It is perfectly reasonable to reassure them that after a significant period of time without any mental health symptoms, they can begin to consider coming off the medicine. However, the decision shouldn't be taken too lightly and should usually be done in conjunction with the doctor. More consideration is given to this question below.

Following up

Once you've started your patient on an SSRI and given them a full explanation of what to expect, it is important to follow them up.

NICE recommends a 2-week follow-up. However, there are a number of options and each option will be more or less suitable, depending on the patient. These are useful principles.

At 1 week

The SSRI is highly unlikely to have had any discernible positive effect. However, at this time, patients who might be suffering side-effects may be struggling. The 1-week review is least used but is suitable for:

- high-risk patients who need regular review for danger of suicidal thoughts
- patients with a 'pill phobia', who will need reassurance about their new medication and may experience a large nocebo effect
- patients with a history of strong side-effects.

At 1 week you will not be able to:

- assess the effectiveness of the SSRI
- determine if the side-effects are reducing.

At 2 weeks

The is probably the most commonly used follow-up time by clinicians. However, there are limitations to the follow-up at 2 weeks. At 2 weeks you will be able to:

- assess side-effects and hopefully judge whether these are reducing with time
- assess whether there has been any dip in mood or worsening of the underlying mental health condition.

However, at 2 weeks, you will not be able to:

- determine if the SSRI is effective at reducing mental health symptoms. For some people there could be some early effect by now; however, it will be impossible to judge lack of effectiveness
- determine if the dose is effective and correct.

At 4 weeks

Four weeks is also a very popular choice for follow-up if the patient is suitable. The 4-week follow-up may be more suitable for:

- patients who are relatively stable and show low risk for suicidal thoughts
- patients who have previously been on an SSRI with no issues.

The 4-week follow-up has a number of advantages:

- the early side-effects should have worn off, so any lingering side-effects could indicate that these may persist longer-term with the medicine
- you can now judge the effectiveness of the medication – for most patients the SSRI will have started to work. This can be a useful time to start to determine dose corrections or medication changes.

The disadvantages of the 4-week follow-up are:

- there has been no earlier check-in, so there is a risk of patient non-adherence if there are side-effects
- higher-risk patients may have deteriorated and safety-netting is less secure.

At 6 weeks

At 6 weeks it can be assumed that the SSRI is now having its full effect, although technically, this may not always be the case as some patients do need to wait longer. However, at this point, it is reasonable to start to make dose adjustments for patients who have responded partially, or switch medication for those that have not responded at all.

Patients can do PHQ-9 or GAD-7 scores before the follow-up meetings, saving time in the consultation.

After the first follow-up

The first follow-up is likely to have been at 1, 2 or 4 weeks. Following this, you should book the next follow-up depending on whether there have been any changes to the medication, whether the patient is showing signs of improvement and the overall suicide risk.

Monitoring and evaluating an SSRI

There is no need to overcomplicate the assessment of the effectiveness of the SSRI.

A good, formal and well-evidenced way to monitor progress is to perform serial PHQ-9 assessments for the patient with depression, or GAD-7 for the patient with anxiety. This can give you a reasonable reference point for the objective monitoring of the patient's progress. This is advisable and recommended by NICE; however, it does require a degree of time investment at each follow-up.

Patients can do PHQ-9 or GAD-7 scores before the follow-up meetings, saving time in the consultation.

A quick and simple way to give you some idea of the balance between positive and negative effects of the drug is to ask the patient to score the drug out of 10 on two questions.

1. Out of 10, how much has the medicine improved your symptoms? 10 out 10 means your mental health condition is completely resolved and you are entirely back to your normal self, and 0 out of 10 means it has done nothing useful at all.
2. Out of 10, was the medicine suitable for not giving you side-effects? 10 out 10 means you experienced absolutely no side-effects, whereas 0 out of 10 means the side-effects were extremely bad and intolerable.

The perfect result is a score of 10 and 10. This is rarely achieved; however, it can help determine your next step. See the table below for suggestions:

Effectiveness score	Side-effect score	Action
Good	Good	Great – little may need to change. You could consider a dose drop – can the same result be achieved with a lower dose?
Good	Poor	The medicine is performing well but with side-effects – consider a dose drop or switch medicine.
Poor	Good	The medicine is well tolerated but ineffective – consider a dose increase. If still no benefit – switch drug.
Poor	Poor	It is unlikely this medicine is going to be useful. If very early, you could wait to see if the effectiveness improves and the side-effects dissipate, but it is likely that a drug change is needed.

Once you have started the SSRI, and have followed that patient up, you will have a number of options at your disposal.

1. Keep the medication the same and follow the patient up again
2. Add the medication to the patient's repeat and stop follow-up
3. Make a dose change and follow the patient up
4. Change the medicine and follow the patient up
5. Stop the medicine and follow the patient up.

You will choose your options based on the effectiveness of the medicine, its side-effect profile and the overall acceptability to the patient of the medicine.

Stopping an SSRI

Many patients will be keen to come off their medicines once they feel better. Generally speaking these times are recommended as a minimum duration of taking them:

- First or second episode of illness – minimum of 6–9 months
- Three or more episodes – minimum of 2 years
- Recurrent illness with multiple relapses – where appropriate, these patients can safely remain on SSRIs lifelong.

A good time to consider stopping an SSRI would be:

- after the minimum duration period
- after a spell of at least 8 weeks with no symptoms of the underlying condition.

There are several reasons to stop an SSRI that are less appropriate:

- The patient has been on the drug 'too long'. There is no maximal length of time that a patient can take an SSRI and if symptoms of the underlying medical condition are still there or very likely to return on cessation, then it is ill-advised to stop.
- The patient has been advised by other people to stop them.
  - this is often a feature of the prejudice and misinformation that is rife in society

- The patient feels stigmatised by them.
  - this is a significant problem and it would be better to address the stigma through education than necessarily stop a useful treatment. Nevertheless, in these cases other treatment options should be considered too.

How to stop them

The length of time required to taper down the antidepressant will depend on its half-life. The SSRI with the shortest half-life is paroxetine and it is therefore associated with the highest likelihood of cessation effects – hence its use has significantly diminished.

Fluoxetine has the longest half-life and has the lowest likelihood of causing discontinuation effects.

When stopping an SSRI, gradually reduce the dose, normally over a 2–4 week period. Bear in mind that some patients will need longer, whilst others manage with less than a week with no ill effects.

Patients should be counselled about discontinuation effects but also to remain vigilant about the recurrence of the underlying mental health condition. If discontinuation effects occur than restart the medicine at a low dose and slow the process of tapering off.

Discontinuation or recurrence of illness?

Discontinuation symptoms can in some cases mimic those of depression or anxiety. The following may help in differentiation:

- Discontinuation effects emerge within days of stopping the medication. Relapse symptoms develop later and more gradually.
- Discontinuation effects often include physical complaints not found in the underlying mental health condition, e.g. dizziness, flu-like symptoms and abnormal sensations.
- Discontinuation effects disappear quickly after taking a dose of the withdrawn SSRI, whilst a recurrence of underlying depression or anxiety can take several weeks to resolve.

- Discontinuation effects improve over days to weeks, whereas a recurrence of mental health illness continues to worsen over time.

SSRIs in pregnancy and breastfeeding

Contrary to common public perception, SSRIs can be taken during pregnancy and breastfeeding. NICE guideline CG192: *Antenatal and postnatal mental health: clinical management and service guidance* can help with this decision-making[16]. As with all medicines used during pregnancy and breastfeeding, a risk and benefit analysis should be done with the patient and you should consult the BNF for advice on an individual drug. However, it is not the case that women must come off an SSRI at the time of pregnancy, or indeed in the postnatal period. A study in the *BMJ* [17] has suggested that on review of SSRIs used in the third trimester reported as causing birth defects, no association could be confirmed for sertraline. Sertraline is also the most commonly used SSRI in the ante- and postnatal period. There remain questions over the association of paroxetine with birth defects and although these involve very small numbers, and could not be confirmed with any statistical significance, it would be advised not to use paroxetine at all.

Many patients, however, are not aware that SSRIs can be continued at all during pregnancy and you may see a number of scenarios:

- Some women will stop the medicine altogether at the time they start planning a pregnancy
- They may stop once they find out they are pregnant
- They may consult with you before stopping in the expectation of starting a family
- They may completely put off pregnancy in the fear that they may need to stop their medicines or risk a deterioration in their mental health.

---

[16] NICE (2014) *Antenatal and postnatal mental health: clinical management and service guidance.* Clinical guideline [CG192].

[17] Reefhuis, J., Devine, O., Friedman, J.M. *et al.* (2015) Specific SSRIs and birth defects: bayesian analysis to interpret new data in the context of previous reports. *BMJ,* **351**:h3190.

It is important that you take your patient through a risk–benefit discussion. Use the following points:

- Women should be encouraged to discuss any changes to their medicines with you before stopping
- No psychotropic medication has a UK marketing authorisation specifically for women who are pregnant or breast-feeding
  - however, SSRIs have been used for many decades and there is very little evidence of harm to the mother or baby
  - some small studies have found a very small incidence of neonatal adjustment syndrome, where the baby shows signs of discontinuation lasting about a week – but this is rare
- There are likely to be risks associated with stopping, including a recurrence of the mental health condition, which could be harmful to the pregnancy or the baby
- Where a cessation of the SSRI is still needed or wanted by the patient:
  - withdraw the medicine slowly
  - offer an alternative such as CBT.

6.5.3 SNRIs

SNRIs are monoamine reuptake inhibitors, in that they inhibit the reuptake of serotonin and noradrenaline. Selective serotonin reuptake inhibitors (SSRIs) act upon serotonin only.

Dual inhibition of serotonin and noradrenaline reuptake is thought to offer several advantages over SSRIs. SNRIs can be especially useful in concomitant chronic or neuropathic pain. SNRIs, along with SSRIs, are second-generation antidepressants.

In 1993, venlafaxine became the first commercially available SNRI.

Some studies have shown that antidepressant drugs which have combined serotonergic and noradrenergic activity are generally more effective than SSRIs, which act upon serotonin reuptake alone. However, the same studies suggest they are, overall, slightly less well tolerated.

SNRIs might have greater pain-relieving properties in comparison to SSRIs. Serotonin and noradrenaline are likely to be involved in the physiology of the pain response. SNRIs may be more suitable in reducing pain and functional impairment in neuropathic pain conditions – especially when associated with a mental health condition. SNRIs have been used to reduce doses of other pain-relieving medication such as opioids. There is a very well-established link between pain and mental health illness and often a failure to treat both can result in improvement in neither.

Duloxetine in particular has been shown to significantly reduce pain-related symptoms of sufferers of generalised anxiety disorder, after short-term and long-term treatment.

Choice of SNRI

Currently there are two SNRIs available in the UK:

- Venlafaxine (since 1993)
- Duloxetine (since 2004)

A further four are available in the USA:

- Sibutramine (since 1998)
- Desvenlafaxine (since 2008)
- Milnacipran (since 2009)
- Levomilnacipran (since 2013).

Why choose an SNRI?

Due to the poorer tolerability and interaction profile of SNRIs, these are considered second-line after SSRIs.

The same consideration should be given to the commencement of an SNRI as that given to an SSRI in terms of patient explanations. They follow a similar pattern of initiation and discontinuation effects and have a similar profile in terms of duration of treatment and time of onset of effects.

SNRIs generally have a shorter half-life than SSRIs and, as previously stated, a shorter half-life can be associated with worse discontinuation effects. They should therefore be tapered off more slowly.

Drug	Half-life (hours)
Venlafaxine	5
Venlafaxine MR	11
Duloxetine	12

Advantages

Some studies suggest that the SNRIs venlafaxine and duloxetine are more effective and work with a quicker onset than SSRIs. However, this advantage is not conclusively proven. For a patient who has not found an SSRI effective, changing to an SNRI may provide a more meaningful switch, rather than side-stepping to another SSRI.

SNRIs, particularly duloxetine, have an association with improvement of neuropathic pain. This can be advantageous in the treatment of patients with fibromyalgia, where the mental health symptoms are accompanied by physical pain.

Disadvantages

- SNRIs are associated with the same range of side-effects as SSRIs.
- SNRIs can produce a sharp increase in non-adrenergic activity shortly after commencement.
- Venlafaxine has a short half-life and so its discontinuation effects may be stronger. You should therefore lower the dose more slowly than would be needed for other SNRIs or SSRIs, on cessation of this drug.
- SNRIs can increase blood pressure and this should be monitored. Blood pressure should ideally be controlled before starting.
- SNRIs are strongly cautioned against in patients with pre-existing coronary heart disease.
- Duloxetine has also been associated with cases of liver failure and should not be prescribed to patients with chronic alcohol use or liver disease.

6.5.4 Tricyclic antidepressants (TCAs)

These were discovered in the early 1950s and are named after their chemical structure, which contains three rings of atoms.

TCAs are considered 'first-generation' antidepressants and for the most part have been superseded by SSRIs (second-generation). Although they are still generally considered to be highly effective, the main reason for replacement by newer antidepressants is an improved safety and side-effect profile. TCAs overall have a higher number of severe side-effects and are also more likely to result in death if used in a suicide attempt, as the doses required for clinical treatment and potentially lethal overdose are relatively close, in comparison to an SSRI.

Tricyclic and related antidepressant drugs can be roughly divided into those with sedative properties and those that are less sedating. Agitated patients may respond best to the sedative TCAs, whereas withdrawn and apathetic patients will often obtain most benefit from the less sedating ones. Sedative TCAs can naturally help with sleep also and should therefore be prescribed at night time. Non-sedating ones can be used during the day, although it should be noted that even these can produce some degree of drowsiness in the day. Trazodone is listed here under TCAs, and whilst related, its pharmacology is more complex and is sometimes considered 'atypical'.

Sedative TCAs:

- Amitriptyline
- Clomipramine
- Dosulepin
- Mianserin
- Trazodone (most sedating)
- Trimipramine.

Less sedative TCAs:

- Imipramine
- Lofepramine
- Nortriptyline.

TCAs for neuropathic pain

It should be noted that many TCAs are used for the treatment of neuropathic pain. The most commonly used for this purpose is amitriptyline. However, whilst amitriptyline has pain-relieving properties at doses as low as 10mg, its antidepressant dose is a much higher 50–75mg as a minimum. Lower doses may not produce much antidepression effect.

TCAs can be used for a number of other indications, such as migraine prophylaxis, and occasionally to induce sleep. The initial dosing for this is 10mg, significantly lower than needed for an antidepressant effect.

Side-effects

One of the main disadvantages of TCAs, and a big reason for the dominance of SSRIs over them, is the range, frequency and severity of side-effects they can produce. These are mainly due to their antimuscarinic effects. These include:

- dry mouth
- dry nose
- blurry vision
- lowered gastrointestinal motility or constipation
- urinary retention
- cognitive impairment
- increased body temperature.

Nevertheless, there are still many patients who can tolerate these drugs well and they can be a helpful second- or third-line option for patients who have failed to respond to an SSRI or an SNRI.

Speed of onset and discontinuation

TCAs can sometimes start to work faster than SSRIs. Their sedating effect is felt within hours. However, for most people, the antidepressant effect can take several weeks, much the same as SSRIs. They can also be associated with discontinuation effects, similar to SSRIs. Since the side-effects can be stronger with TCAs, it is advisable to titrate the dose up more slowly in the initiation phase and reduce more slowly in the discontinuation phase.

Why would you switch to a TCA?

TCAs are first-generation drugs and have largely been superseded. However, they may have a role to play:

- as a third-line agent for patients who fail to respond to SSRIs or SNRIs
- for patients who need sedation (e.g. to help sleep)
- for patients who also have a need to treat neuropathic pain.

Which one to choose?

Lofepramine has a lower incidence of side-effects and is less dangerous in overdosage; it is considered by NICE to be the TCA of choice if it is to be used for depression.

Imipramine is often reported to have much more marked anti-muscarinic side-effects than other tricyclics.

Amitriptyline and **dosulepin** are effective but they are particularly dangerous in overdosage and are not recommended for the treatment of depression. NICE recommends that dosulepin should be initiated by a specialist and in general this drug is not recommended for use in primary care due to its cardiotoxicity – particularly in the elderly.

Trazodone is the most sedating and is used sometimes, in particular to help with agitated patients. It is safer to use this than antipsychotics in elderly patients who need pharmacological sedation for confusion, aggression, agitation or delirium.

6.5.5 Atypical antidepressants

Mirtazapine

Mirtazapine is a noradrenergic and specific serotonergic anti-depressant (NaSSA); it does not have effects as a monoamine reuptake inhibitor. It also has a significant effect at the histamine 1 receptor, making it sleep-inducing and causing weight gain.

Mirtazapine has no significant drug–drug interactions; this makes it attractive for use in combination with other antidepressants as an augmenting option – usually with an SSRI or SNRI.

Side-effects, initiation and discontinuation

The side-effect profile is not dissimilar to SSRIs; however, the following differences are clinically relevant:

- It is more likely to cause weight gain through an increase in appetite
- It is more likely to cause sedation (in fact it is often chosen for this property); however, patients may experience drowsiness the following morning

- It is LESS associated with sexual dysfunction side-effects in comparison to SSRIs
- It is LESS associated with nausea and tremor.

Mirtazapine should be considered a drug that has a similar initiation and discontinuation effect and time period as SSRIs, although individual patients can differ in their personal experience.

Mirtazapine is not an addictive substance.

Why would I choose mirtazapine?

Mirtazapine can be considered as a single agent, or in combination with another drug such as an SSRI or SNRI:

- in patients who have a need for night-time sedation, i.e. those with long-term insomnia
- in patients who have sexual dysfunction with SSRI or SNRIs
- in patients who have not responded to first-line treatments
- in combination with another drug (SSRI or SNRI) and as an adjunct for patients who have only partially responded.

6.5.6 Benzodiazepines

A brief history

The first benzodiazepine produced was chlordiazepoxide in 1955 by Hoffmann–La Roche. As is often the case, the compound was found accidentally. A crystalline substance was found left over from an abandoned project while spring-cleaning in the lab. Researchers submitted it for a standard battery of tests, more in hope than expectation, but found it showed very strong sedative, anticonvulsant and muscle relaxant effects. The marketing was fast throughout the world and in 1960 it was released under the brand name Librium. Diazepam, also created by Hoffmann–La Roche (under the name Valium), was released in 1963. These were both extremely successful, from a commercial point of view, for the parent company.

Prior to the introduction of benzodiazepines, the main drugs used for anxiety and sedation were barbiturates; in comparison benzodiazepines were much more effective and better tolerated. By the 1970s they had almost completely replaced the older drugs and by 1977 they were the single most prescribed drug globally.

At the time, the risk of dependence was not known, or at least not acknowledged. In fact, one of the key advertised advantages was the lower chance of addiction in comparison to barbiturates. However, by 1980 it was clear that these drugs were strongly associated with addiction, tolerance, dependence and withdrawal.

Benzodiazepines became the subject of the largest ever class-action lawsuit against drug manufacturers in the UK, involving tens of thousands of patients alleging that the manufacturers knew of the dependence potential but intentionally withheld this information from doctors. Hundreds of GPs and health authorities were also sued by individual patients.

The court case against the drug manufacturers, costing over £30 million, never reached a verdict and fell through. This story of a new drug, brought fast to market, creating addiction amongst potentially hundreds of thousands of people before being reclassified and properly labelled as addictive, has undoubtedly played its part in the concern, suspicion and fear that many patients to this day have about any medicine involved in the treatment of a mental health disorder. Many younger patients will tell of a parent or another family member a generation or two older than them who was addicted to antidepressants, and often that drug would have been a benzodiazepine. It is a common reason for the patient not wishing to go down 'that route' of treatment for their illness.

Currently available benzodiazepines

There are over a dozen different generic benzodiazepines available. They have strong recreational and abuse potential and as such can easily be found through unregulated and criminal sources.

They are generally subdivided into short- and long-acting. Common examples of both types are as follows:

Short-acting (half-life approx. 2-12 hours)

- Alprazolam
- Lorazepam
- Oxazepam
- Temazepam.

Long-acting (half-life approx. 20-100 hours)

- Nitrazepam
- Diazepam
- Chlordiazepoxide.

Indications for use

Benzodiazepines are not indicated for use in anxiety, depression or other mental health disorders for anything other than short-term relief of significant agitation or sleeplessness. There should be a clear case made for their use which should include:

- the fact that the patient is in significant distress which needs an immediate intervention
- the symptoms will be short-lived and likely to have some natural end.

An example of appropriate use would be a patient who has just started on an SSRI who you know will need to wait several weeks to get an effect, who is also showing extreme anxiety, agitation or sleeplessness. In this patient, there is an immediate need, and a reason to believe that the symptoms will improve once the SSRI starts to work.

Another example might be short-term insomnia after a traumatic event such as a burglary. The patient has insomnia of recent onset, clearly provoked by a life event. It is likely that after a short time the insomnia will settle and a very short course of benzodiazepines may suffice.

In a patient with chronic insomnia, the strategy of using a benzodiazepine is inappropriate.

Despite the fact that this class of drug should not be used long-term, its benefits in the short term should not be overlooked or dismissed. Patients who are showing strong signs of distress can be reassured that the short-term use of a drug like diazepam, in association with a better longer-term strategy, can be appropriate and hugely beneficial to the right patient.

Side-effects

Benzodiazepines are associated with short- and long-term side-effects:

- Sedation and muscle relaxation
- Dizziness
- Reduced concentration and coordination (impaired ability to drive)

- Risk of falls (especially in the elderly)
- Disinhibition.

Long-term effects

- **Tolerance** – the need to continually increase the dose to achieve the same effect as previously achieved with a lower dose. After 4–6 months, the drug may produce no discernible effect with a prolonged break from it.
- **Dependence rebound and withdrawal** – rebound is the return of the symptoms for which the patient was treated, but worse than before. Withdrawal symptoms are the new symptoms that occur when the benzodiazepine is stopped. They are the main sign of physical dependence.

For these reasons, benzodiazepines should not be used for longer than a few weeks at most.

Discontinuation

Whilst SSRIs can be associated with a discontinuation syndrome which is present in relatively few people and relatively easily tempered with a 2–4 week dose reduction before stopping, benzodiazepines that have been used long-term are significantly more difficult to stop.

They should not be stopped abruptly. The patient must be informed of the benefits of stopping or reducing and it is vital that they 'buy in' to this – much like smoking cessation. The drug will normally have to be withdrawn over many months and this can even be years but with good support from the clinician it is perfectly possible to achieve. It might be anticipated that for a small minority of patients, this cannot be done and some patients may require the help of addiction services.

6.5.7 Non-benzodiazepine hypnotics (Z-drugs)

These are a class of psychoactive drugs that are very benzodiazepine-like in nature. They are used in the treatment of sleep problems. Originally thought to be less addictive and withdrawal-inducing than benzodiazepines, these drugs have been shown to be both addictive and the subject of abuse.

As such they should be used with the same precaution as benzo-diazepines.

Current drugs

- Zolpidem
- Zopiclone
- Zaleplon (rarely prescribed in the UK).

Side-effects

- Taste disturbance (some report a metallic-like taste)
- Nausea, vomiting
- Next day sedation (these drugs have been associated with motor vehicle accidents)
- Dry mouth
- Rarely, amnesia.

Why would I use them?

These drugs are only indicated for very short-term insomnia and you should be assured that the symptoms are likely to be short-lived. They are sometimes used to augment the initiation of an SSRI, with the sleep likely to improve once the SSRI began to work a few weeks after starting.

Short-term sleep problems associated with a traumatic event may also be a reasonable use case. The patient should be counselled that they can produce dependence and are not appropriate for repeat prescribing.

Patients who have been on these long-term may need the same support as those taking benzodiazepines in a slow, controlled and supported cessation.

6.5.8 Antihistamines as hypnotics

H1-antihistamines are compounds that inhibit the activity of the H1 receptor and are obviously used to treat allergic reactions, amongst other conditions. First-generation antihistamines have a tendency to cross the blood–brain barrier and as such can cause sedation. Second-generation antihistamines (non-drowsy) do not do so. These older antihistamines such as diphenhydramine and promethazine are therefore used to treat insomnia. Most hay fever and allergy remedies sold in pharmacies will now use non-drowsy second-generation antihistamines.

The drugs are readily available over the counter in pharmacies.

Commonly available drugs

- Diphenhydramine (e.g. Nytol) – available OTC
- Promethazine – available OTC
- Hydroxyzine.

Why would I use these?

Whilst there is some evidence that diphenhydramine can cause a very mild case of dependence in some people, antihistamines are not generally considered a drug associated with addiction and withdrawal. However, tolerance to the sleep-inducing effect is well-documented.

Antihistamines of this type can be suggested for patients with short-term sleep problems where the patient has tried basic sleep hygiene measures and these have failed. It is a much safer option than the prescription hypnotics described above but overall their power and effect will be noticeably milder. Nevertheless, a majority of patients will notice a clinical benefit in their ability to get off to sleep, and maintain sleep through the night. Caution should be advised for 'morning after' drowsiness effects.

6.5.9 Monoamine oxidase inhibitors

Monoamine oxidase inhibitors (MAOIs) are a class of drugs that inhibit the activity of one or both monoamine oxidase enzymes: monoamine oxidase A or B. The original drugs were 'non-reversible' inhibitors but there are more modern drugs that are 'reversible'. They have in the past been shown to have a high efficacy as antidepressants. However, their use has diminished significantly over the last half-century. This is primarily due to their potential for interaction with other drugs and their potential for interaction with some dietary substances – notably those containing tyramine, which is found in products such as cheese, soy sauce and salami. They have been implicated in the development of severe hypertension and the fatal serotonin syndrome in patients.

This potential for serious interaction with a number of substances – including common food items – has led to the almost complete discontinuation of this class of drug for use in depression or anxiety. Non-reversible MAOIs, such as phenelzine, should be prescribed only by specialist mental health professionals and are rarely seen nowadays.

Reversible inhibitor of monoamine oxidase (RIMA)

The drug moclobemide is a RIMA. Unlike the older non-reversible MAOIs, this drug does not display the dangerous interaction with tyramine in food substances; hence it is considered safer. Some trials have suggested it is at least equally as efficacious as TCAs and SSRIs, with a similar tolerability profile. Moclobemide was found, unlike most other antidepressants on the market, to actually improve all aspects of sexual function.

Nevertheless, it still has drawbacks and cautions such as possible drug–drug interaction and a dangerous interaction with general anaesthesia, making it a difficult drug to prescribe. Initiation in primary care is ill-advised; however, it is useful to know about it and have some understanding of its place.

6.5.10 Pregabalin and gabapentin

Pregabalin and the older gabapentin are anticonvulsant and anxiolytic medications used to treat epilepsy, neuropathic pain, fibromyalgia, restless leg syndrome and anxiety disorders.

NICE suggests that pregabalin can be offered as a second-line agent to patients who have failed to respond to SSRIs or SNRIs. It can also be used as an adjunct to other drugs such as SSRIs.

Pregabalin is moderately effective and is safe for treatment of generalised anxiety disorder. It appears to have anxiolytic effects similar to benzodiazepines, with less risk of dependence.

The effects of pregabalin appear more quickly than SSRIs but a little less quickly than benzodiazepines – with maximal effect visible after about one week of use. Pregabalin has demonstrated superiority by producing more consistent therapeutic effects for psychosomatic anxiety symptoms. It is generally not thought to elicit much tolerance effect – in other words, doses don't have to be increased just to achieve the same effect with time. It has a beneficial effect on sleep. It produces less severe cognitive and psychomotor impairment compared to benzodiazepines.

A 2019 review[18] found that pregabalin reduces symptoms, and was generally well tolerated.

Side-effects

- Weight gain
- Sleepiness and fatigue
- Dizziness and vertigo
- Leg swelling
- Disturbed vision
- Loss of coordination
- Euphoria.

Cautions

Abrupt discontinuation of pregabalin can result in symptoms suggestive of physical dependence. The overall profile of pregabalin is such that it is considered less addictive than benzodiazepines. However, even people who have discontinued short-term use of pregabalin have experienced withdrawal symptoms, including insomnia, headache and flu-like illness.

Pregabalin is considered a drug with abuse potential and can be found through illicit means on the black market. Clinicians should be mindful of this.

Why would I use pregabalin?

Pregabalin can be considered a third-line agent, or an adjunctive ther-

---

[18] Slee, A., Nazareth, I., Bondaronek, P. *et al.* (2019) Pharmacological treatments for generalised anxiety disorder: a systematic review and network meta-analysis. *Lancet*, **393(10173):** 768–777.

apy to those patients already on an SSRI but without good response. In the UK, pregabalin is classified as a Class C controlled drug.

It does have abuse and addiction potential so clinicians should be mindful of this. Patients with a history of dependence may be less suitable candidates.

6.5.11 Buspirone

Buspirone acts as an agonist of the serotonin 5-HT receptor, although its full action in relation to its anxiolytic effects is not fully known. It is used for the short-term treatment of anxiety disorders or symptoms of anxiety. It is generally less preferred to SSRIs and it is used little in the UK; however, it is more popular in the USA.

Buspirone has a delayed action for its anxiolytic effects, similar to SSRIs, of about 2–4 weeks before full clinical effectiveness. It has also been used as an adjunct to SSRIs, although evidence is limited and NICE does not recommend this.

It has a similar side-effect profile to the SNRIs. This drug is rarely used in primary care in the UK.

Buspirone has been trialled in the treatment of hypoactive sexual desire disorder with some limited success. It was also tried, unsuccessfully, as a treatment for benzodiazepine and alcohol withdrawal.

It may be preferable to SSRIs and SNRIs for those with significant side-effects.

6.5.12 Beta-blockers

Beta-blockers have multiple uses, e.g. the management of abnormal heart rhythms, secondary prevention after myocardial infarction and the treatment of high blood pressure.

They are competitive antagonists that block the receptor sites for the endogenous catecholamines adrenaline and noradrenaline, therefore inhibiting the sympathetic nervous system, which mediates the 'flight or fight' response.

Since beta-receptors are found on cells of the heart muscles, smooth muscles, airways, arteries, kidneys, and other tissues that are part of the sympathetic nervous system, beta-blockers can have a wide range of physiological effects on the body. The discovery of beta-blockers is considered by some as one of the most important contributions to clinical medicine of the 20th century.

Beta-blockers have no psychotropic effects and therefore will not impact on any of the cognitive symptoms of anxiety. Their role is simply to control the 'downstream' adrenergic symptoms produced in patients when they are suffering from an anxiety-mediated panic attack. Some people have used them for performance-related anxiety, such as musical performers who need to reduce the adrenaline effect before a stage performance without inducing the sedation effects associated with benzodiazepines.

Side-effects

- Tiredness
- Dizziness or light-headedness (secondary to bradycardia)
- Cold fingers or toes (exacerbation of Raynaud's syndrome)
- Difficulties sleeping or nightmares
- Nausea.

Time of onset

Beta-blockers have a fast period of onset. They will produce effects within a few hours. Depending on the formulation, the effect can last from 6–24 hours. For this reason some people have used them as a 'pill in the pocket' approach to stopping panic attacks. Some CBT practitioners, however, feel this approach limits the patient's ability to respond behaviourally to panic symptoms and can hinder their overall recovery.

Why would I use a beta-blocker?

Remember that beta-blockers have no impact on the cognitive and emotional effects of depression or anxiety and as such are not psychotropic antidepressants or anxiolytics per se. They do, however, successfully blockade the sympathetic nervous system and can therefore help with the adrenergic symptoms experienced by patients with anxiety and panic disorders. This may have some benefit on 'secondary' anxiety, which is the cognitive anxiety induced after feedback from physical symptoms. In effect, they stop the vicious circle of the mind racing, followed by the heart racing, followed by the mind racing.

6.5.13 Antipsychotics

Antipsychotics, also known as neuroleptics, are used to manage psychosis, principally in schizophrenia but also in a range of other psychiatric disorders – including depression with psychosis, bipolar disorder and generalised anxiety disorder. Some of these uses are off-licence. Antipsychotics can be used to augment other drugs such as SSRIs.

The initiation of antipsychotics in primary care is not advised and NICE makes this clear in its guidance on depression and anxiety. Nevertheless, within primary care, you will see patients on these drugs and it is useful to have a good grasp of them.

Current antipsychotics

First-generation (abbreviated list)

- Haloperidol
- Chlorpromazine
- Levomepromazine
- Prochlorperazine
- Flupentixol.

Second-generation – atypical (abbreviated list)

- Lurasidone
- Risperidone
- Aripiprazole
- Olanzapine
- Quetiapine.

The second-generation antipsychotic quetiapine is probably the most commonly used adjunct for major depressive disorder in combination with an SSRI.

Side-effects

- Involuntary movement disorders
- Gynaecomastia
- Impotence

- Weight gain
- Metabolic syndrome
- Long-term use – tardive dyskinesia.

Why would I use an antipsychotic?

Patients with symptoms of psychosis should all be managed in secondary care. These drugs should be initiated in secondary care. In primary care, you will come across them and should be aware of their issues and adverse effects.

6.5.14 Combinations and drug augmentation

A significant proportion of adult patients newly diagnosed with major depression or anxiety do not achieve complete relief of symptoms after taking one antidepressant. These remission rates apply to both first- and second-generation antidepressants such as SSRIs.

Whilst the option of dose increases is a natural first step, there is also an option to combine or augment the medication. A number of these combinations have been studied and are suggested by NICE in certain circumstances. NICE does, however, recommend that these combinations should only be initiated in primary care after some discussion with a psychiatrist.

Augmentation is generally considered an option only when a first drug provides partial relief but does not completely alleviate symptoms. This could, however, increase the likelihood of side-effects and drug interactions.

One of the most relevant studies for real-world clinical practice, the Sequenced Treatment Alternatives to Relieve Depression (STAR*D) trial[19], found that both psychotherapy and drugs are about equally effective as augmentation strategies.

Some combinations

It is possible to combine different classes of antidepressant medi-

[19] National Institute of Mental Health (NIMH) (2002) *Sequenced Treatment Alternatives to Relieve Depression (STAR*D) research protocol.* Revised ed. NIMH.

cines to produce a possible augmented benefit. However, from NICE guidelines, be aware of the following points:

- Select medications that are known to be safe when used together.
- Be mindful of the increased side-effect burden this usually causes.
- You should discuss the rationale for any combination with the person with depression, follow GMC guidance if off-label medication is prescribed, and monitor carefully for adverse effects.
- It is good to know and understand primary evidence and consider obtaining a second opinion when using unusual combinations, if the evidence for the efficacy of a chosen strategy is limited or the risk–benefit ratio is unclear.
- People who have had multiple episodes of depression and who have a good response to augmentation should remain on this treatment if side-effects are acceptable.
- Once improvement is recorded, if one medication is stopped, it should usually be the augmenting agent.

SSRI or SNRI + mirtazapine

Adding mirtazapine as an adjunct to an SSRI or SNRI, e.g. venla-faxine + mirtazapine, is considered a pharmacologically safe option and was studied in the STAR*D trial. Patients may report a higher side-effect burden but the study did show a small but significant overall improvement in remission rate for previously resistant depression patients.

Mirtazapine is generally considered a more appropriate adjunct than lithium or an antipsychotic, as it does not interact with other antidepressant classes.

SSRI + lithium

Most primary care clinicians would feel that it is outside their scope of expertise to initiate lithium. However, lithium can be used to augment a number of classes of antidepressant, including SSRIs.

NICE recommends that when using lithium the clinician should:

- monitor renal and thyroid function before treatment and every 6 months during treatment (more often if there is evidence of renal impairment)
- consider ECG monitoring in people with depression who are at high risk of cardiovascular disease
- monitor serum lithium levels 1 week after initiation and each dose change until stable, and every 3 months thereafter.

SSRI or SNRI + antipsychotic

As with lithium, most primary care clinicians will feel that initiating an antipsychotic is outside their expertise. Patients showing signs of psychosis should always be referred into secondary care; however, even without psychosis, patients with drug-resistant depression can use antipsychotics as augmenters.

The most common antipsychotics used are quetiapine, risperidone and aripiprazole. When a patient is augmented with such a drug, NICE recommends monitoring of weight, lipid and glucose levels, and side-effects (for example, extrapyramidal side-effects and prolactin-related side-effects with risperidone).

6.5.15 Suggested sequencing

The sequence of pharmacological interventions will depend on a number of factors. If the patient has described a clear benefit from a particular medicine in the past then this should be suggested early in the sequence.

If the patient has previously tried a medicine and not described a benefit or described side-effects, then this drug should be considered less suitable. However, you should check that:

- the medicine was used for a sufficient length of time before deciding it is ineffective (usually at least 6 weeks)
- it is used at a sufficiently high dose to determine its effectiveness or ineffectiveness

- side-effects were likely from this drug and not other causes.

As per NICE, the usual starting drug for a range of mental health conditions will be an SSRI. The choice of SSRI has been studied extensively, with many published papers. There is little definitive consensus; however, the majority of practitioners will choose the following based on known levels of general effectiveness, tolerability and cost. Paroxetine should not be used; however, for patients who are already on this drug and are finding it effective with no side-effects, it is unnecessary to change it. What follows is a suggested step-wise sequencing and escalation of pharmacological treatments – but note that there will be many individual factors to consider with the patient in front of you.

Step 1

Basic SSRIs

- Sertraline
- Citalopram
- Escitalopram
- Fluoxetine

Titrate to an effective dose – use BNF as a guide for individual drug dose.

For a patient who has used these medicines, and has found them ineffective (even after dose titration), consider switching in a 'sideways' step first to another first-line SSRI from the list above. However, avoid multiple 'sideways' steps. If more than one first-line SSRI has failed, consider moving to another step. If, however, the reason for the change is an issue of side-effects and tolerability in a patient who is otherwise finding the medicine effective, it may be worth trying a third basic SSRI.

Step 2

SNRIs

- Venlafaxine
- Duloxetine

or

Higher-potency SSRI

- Vortioxetine

or

Atypical antidepressant

- Mirtazapine

Titrate to an effective dose.

A number of options are suggested above for those patients who have failed to respond to a basic SSRI and rather than making further sideways steps, consider moving up onto one of the options above. There may be specific pros and cons of each, which are described under their own sections (e.g. mirtazapine may be more suitable for patients complaining of sexual dysfunction with other meds).

Step 3

Tricyclic antidepressants

- Lofepramine (generally best tolerated)
- Amitriptyline (most dangerous in overdose)
- Trazodone (most sedating)

Titrate to an effective dose.

TCAs may be tried next; however, it should be noted that this class of drug has disadvantages in comparison to SSRIs and SNRIs – most notably the extra potential side-effects and the much higher risk of harm from overdose. Nevertheless, there remain patients who respond to these older medicines who fail to respond to newer ones.

Step 4

Combinations and augmentations

- SSRI or SNRI in combination with
  - mirtazapine

- ○ lithium
- ○ antipsychotics.

NICE recommends a secondary care opinion before embarking on augmentation therapy and most primary care clinicians would find it outside their scope of expertise. However, augmentation with mirtazapine is probably the most commonly used.

It should be noted that the side-effect risk will go up with the escalating steps described above, and whilst the numbers of patients achieving remission will go up, the returns diminish with each step.

Chapter 7

Summary

Mental health consultations are common in primary care. You will have done many of these, and will continue to do them throughout your clinical career.

These consultations can also be the toughest, in the sense that they take longer, require more emotional resilience and have many obstacles which are not always prevalent in consultations about other illnesses.

Many clinicians are trained in a way which lends itself well to the diagnosing and treating of illnesses which have clear definitions and are generally understood by the public at large. Many people have a concept of what cancer is or what diabetes is. Most clinicians can help their patients with any gaps in their knowledge or understanding of these illnesses through careful discussion. However, mental illnesses often do not have a universally understood meaning and they are shrouded in misconception and stigma. Many people still do not even believe in the existence of such things – they suggest depression is simply a personality flaw.

When trying to offer treatment to a patient suffering from such an illness, who has such misapprehensions, your consultation will need much more time to overcome this. A big part of the problem is the invisibility of mental illness, and the 'short circuit' is a simple and intuitive way of visualising this invisible illness and removing some of the stigma associated with mental illness.

I hope that the ideas and methods described in this book can help overcome these issues and give you and your patient a better consultation experience.

7.1 Visualising mental illness

Chapter 2 has described the normal 'train of thought' through the mind in a logical workflow with an end-point, and differentiated it from the flow of thought in a patient with a condition such as anxiety or depression where the train of thought now 'short circuits'. This can then be represented, visually, on a simple diagram.

Visualising mental illness in this way has a number of advantages. First, it becomes more real, tangible and describable. It is now something people can relate to in the way they are feeling and thinking.

Giving the mental illness a specific identity and tangible description helps separate the illness from an individual's sense of self. They can now point at a diagram and say, 'life problems are represented here, my personality is represented here, and this separate bit is the mental illness – this is the pathology'.

By referring to this simple 'circuit diagram' you can see how different types of mental illness, such as anxiety or depression, can be considered almost the same thing. However, with small changes in the nature of the trapped thought, the outward symptoms of the patient can be vastly different. This can be very helpful in explaining to people how these seemingly very different conditions are strongly linked and can therefore be treated with a very similar set of interventions.

The chapter concluded with how the three Ps – personality, pressure and pathology – can be, and are often, confused with each other. Many patients with a treatable pathology live long parts of their life misinterpreting their difficulties as a defect in their personality or an inevitable reaction to a set of life circumstances. By recognising these confusions, you can help more people come to terms with a mental illness and get them treatment sooner rather than later. This will help improve the consultation for both you and your patient.

7.2 Practical advice

Chapter 3 gives you practical advice on the use of the short circuit as a consultation tool.

Section 3.1 has given you a summary of how the short circuit tool can be used in the flow of a consultation process. Mental health consultations are complicated by the presence of stigma and misconception and these can therefore can offer significant resistance to achieving a good and effective treatment plan for your patient.

The short circuit tool helps you get past this. Once you have used the tool, you can go back to offer your patient a very well-evidenced and personalised treatment plan in partnership with the patient.

Sections 3.2 and *3.3* have described two things:

1. **When** to use the short circuit tool
2. **How** to use the short circuit tool in a consultation.

7.2.1 When to use the tool

The short circuit tool can be used in a number of scenarios but is particularly useful when there are misconceptions of the pathology of mental illness. These misconceptions can take a number of forms. Using the three Ps model, they can be broken down into a few common forms:

1. Pathology confused with personality
2. Pathology confused with pressure.

In *Chapter 3*, you have seen how to look for cues for each of these scenarios and once a cue is noted in a consultation, it may be appropriate to start the short circuit tool.

7.2.2 How to use the tool

Section 3.3 has given you a practical approach to delivering the short circuit tool in a busy consultation. The important thing to remember is that you will develop your own style around it. You will also take more time over certain parts, depending on your individual patient's needs.

This delivery should be practised, bringing it down to a few minutes. When this is done well and engagingly, giving the patient time to take in the information and ask questions, you may have succeeded in removing a lifetime of stigma and misconception for the patient. This is highly likely to make future consultations easier and more productive.

7.3 Mental health in detail

Whilst the short circuit tool can be used to overcome blocks in the consultation relating to stigma and misconception, you will need to have a good understanding of the very common mental illnesses seen in primary care. The sections in these chapters cover epidemiology, presentation, symptoms, diagnosis, causes and treatment options for:

- anxiety (*Section 4.1*)
- depression (*Section 4.2*)
- OCD (*Section 4.3*).

These are extremely common presentations in general practice, and indeed in many secondary care settings. It is important to have a good grasp of these conditions to practise well. Further details on the treatment options are given in *Chapter 6: Treating the patient*.

These sections have also indicated how the short circuit tool can complement the patient's understanding of what is being treated. Remember, the short circuit tool itself should not be used to form a diagnosis or treatment plan. Rather, it should be used to aid the consultation, break stigma and address misconception.

You should then be able to use the usual tools in your armoury to make a diagnosis and offer treatment options.

7.4 Mental health with physical health

Chapter 5 discusses a number of syndromes which have distinct associations with common mental health conditions. Having any of the syndromes described in this chapter is not the same thing as having a diagnosis of a mental health disorder such as depression or anxiety.

However, the syndromes very often coexist and are interlinked with mental illness. The investigation and management of these health conditions requires an exploration of mental health. Indeed, many times the same treatment options can be helpful in the treatment of, for example, IBS and anxiety. Often, exacerbations in one condition lead to exacerbations in the other.

The sections in these chapters have covered epidemiology, presentation, symptoms, diagnosis, causes and treatment options for:

- fibromyalgia (*Section 5.2*)
- irritable bowel syndrome (*Section 5.3*)
- chronic pain syndrome (*Section 5.4*)
- chronic fatigue syndrome (*Section 5.5*).

In particular, the sections have stressed the importance of coexistence of a mental health disorder and the importance of its exploration and management when dealing with these syndromes.

By being able to show your patient neatly, quickly and intuitively how these are intertwined, you will improve their understanding and improve the flow of the consultation.

7.5 Treatments

Chapter 6 has given you an account of the main treatment options available to you to offer your patient. Many common mental health conditions share the same set of pharmacological and non-pharmacological management options. The short circuit does not advocate one treatment over another, but it does allow you to get to this part of the consultation by overcoming the stigma and apprehension that often blocks many consultations from ever getting to this point.

It is important to be able to describe the advantages and disadvantages of each of these treatment modalities and be aware of the high level of stigma, preconception and misconception associated with each. Without adequate explanation of the treatments, patients are more like to be non-compliant. Treatments may not meet patients' preconceived expectations and therefore they may consider treatments a failure before giving them long enough.

As well as having a good grasp of the pharmacology, something many doctors do well, it is important also to understand the concept of talking therapies – and in particular CBT. Misconceptions exist around the nature of this intervention too and many people will resist it on the basis of incorrect information. CBT has a great deal of evidence to support its use and a good consultation should ensure that the patient leaves with a good grasp of the options available to them. They are then much more likely to engage with treatments, have valid expectations of the outcome and feel part of the decision-making process.

7.6 Wrapping up

I sincerely hope that this book has given you tools to tackle some very common problems encountered in primary care consultations. Whilst this won't change your management and diagnosis of mental health conditions, you will, I hope, be able to get through to countless patients who are suffering from a treatable condition for whom stigma and misunderstanding prevent them ever addressing the illness.

There are many examples in medicine of where misinformation clouds an individual's judgement. Hormone replacement therapy, for example, has a perception for many members of the public of a much greater risk of breast cancer than is true. Many people will therefore make a judgement on its relative risk and benefit to themselves on the basis of flawed information.

The erroneous suggestion of a link between the MMR vaccine and autism, first made in the late 1990s, has produced a lasting impression on some people despite irrefutable evidence to show that the original research was flawed, and indeed fraudulent, and there is no link with autism. This is another example of how public perception has influenced a medical decision – in this case the decision of a parent to vaccinate their child.

A good consultation will not have the clinician tell the patient what to do. Moreover, the clinician will give the patient a clear understanding of the benefits and risks of any course of action, with a recommendation, so that the patient can make an informed choice based on good quality information rather than imperfect preconceptions. Helping the patient understand a complex concept in a short period of time is difficult. Whilst skills and techniques to achieve this are rarely taught, the clinician will often have to call upon exactly these skills to aid a good consultation.

The short circuit, used as a consultation tool, provides you with a technique to do this for mental health encounters. Every clinician will have their own consultation style and patter and you will probably develop your own slant on it. My strong recommendation is that you practise it with your peers and colleagues and then try it with patients. With time, this will become a very quick and instinctive thing to do and your consultations will become quicker and more rewarding and the patient will be able to overcome any associated stigma, leading them to a healthy understanding of mental health as a pathology and able to engage better with any treatments.